# CLINICAL PROCEDURES

## Second Edition

# CLINICAL PROCEDURES

## Second Edition

A Concise Guide for
Students of Medicine

## Jack Fisher, M.D., F.A.C.S.
Professor of Surgery
University of California, San Diego, California

## Thomas L. Wachtel, M.D., F.A.C.S.
Associate Professor of Surgery
University of California, San Diego, California

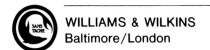

**WILLIAMS & WILKINS**
Baltimore/London

Copyright ©, 1980
The Williams & Wilkins Company
428 E. Preston Street
Baltimore, Md. 21202, U.S.A.

*Made in the United States of America*

Reprinted 1981

Library of Congress Cataloging in Publication Data

Fisher, Jack C          1937–
    Clinical procedures.

    Includes index.
    1. Medicine, Clinical. I. Wachtel, Thomas L., joint author. II. Title.
[DNLM: 1. Diagnosis. 2. Medicine. 3. Physician—Patient relations. WB100
F534c]
RC48.F56 1980        616        80-11509
ISBN 0-683-03240-2

Composed and printed at the
Waverly Press, Inc.
Mt. Royal and Guilford Aves.
Baltimore, Md. 21202, U.S.A.

DEDICATED TO

# THE PATIENT

WHO STANDS TO BENEFIT
MOST FROM THE CONTENT
OF THIS BOOK

# Preface to the Second Edition

A decade has passed since publication of the first edition of Clinical Procedures, a gratifying success which confirmed a conviction that an unfulfilled need did exist. During that interval, the potential audience for a basic primer on clinical skills has enlarged, not just because medical school classes have expanded by nearly 50%, but also because a diverse array of health professionals have become involved in bedside techniques. This trend was not overlooked in the initial preface nor in the selection of topics covered; but knowledge of our current audience has influenced the expansion of this handbook's content.

New subjects include Pelvic Examination, Ventilator Management, and the performance of an Electrocardiographic tracing. Many more chapters required updating; basic patient skills are simply not a timeless body of knowledge! For example, catheter techniques must include Swan-Ganz Catheter insertion and interpretation, thoracostomy must consider use of the Pleurevac, but without abandoning understanding of the classic bottles for water seal drainage. So there is much new along with numerous old and largely unchanged principles. And there are even more illustrations thanks to Julie Hernley and Bill Eckert, our illustrators. Williams & Wilkins has proven themselves a source of continuing support and motivation which characterizes its long-standing medical publishing tradition. Jim Sangston first accepted the concept for edition number one, and here he is again, the force behind a new, improved, more compact, edition number two.

Finally, the reader cannot overlook the dual authorship which assures for this edition a broader perspective. We the authors are also grateful to Doctors William A. Scaring, Thomas K. Butterfield, L. Andrew Rauscher, Hugh A. Frank, John L. Ninnemann, A. Gerson Greenburg, Eugene F. Bernstein, William Bernstein, Richard M. Peters, Ross Rudolph, Joseph D. Schmidt, Lawrence F. Marshall and Sidney L. Saltzstein who checked both facts and opinions, keeping us honest at all times. We are also indebted to Carolyn King, Vera Hobson and Pat Fisher for their clerical and editorial help.

May the patient benefit most, and may all health professionals learn to accept the importance of even the simplest of these procedures.

JACK C. FISHER, M.D.
THOMAS L. WACHTEL, M.D.

# Preface to the First Edition

During his medical education, the student passes through a number of transition zones. Not the least of these occurs at the end of the second year of medical school when he emerges from the classroom and laboratory (with which he has been familiar for many years) and enters an entirely new learning environment, the hospital, where he will be expected to participate in the care of the ill while he learns.

At this stage of training, he has gained a strong foundation of knowledge in the basic medical sciences upon which future clinical training will be built. Achieving this level of proficiency has required a not inconsiderable investment of both time and study. Now, at the beginning of his clinical clerkship, the medical student will be expected to perform a wide variety of basic procedures at the patient's bedside. The preclinical years yield little or no time to discuss these practical skills, and so it falls the lot of the busy house officer to convey his practical knowledge to the student, but only when time permits. Thus, medical students must often acquire manual skills on a trial and error basis with limited supervision ... or they may not learn some procedures at all, leaving them ill-prepared for internship. It is this void which I hope will be partially filled by this small book.

No one would expect a student to learn techniques simply by reading about them, but it is also true that he cannot adequately master a procedure without knowing its physiologic basis, variations, and potential hazards. This volume includes several basic procedures, usually performed at the bedside, which are common to the clinical services a student is exposed to during his clinical clerkship. Advanced techniques peculiar to individual specialties are purposely omitted. Some topics might be considered too advanced for the student, e.g. tracheostomy, but they are included nonetheless so that he might be introduced to them at an early stage of training. Emphasis has been placed on preparation, equipment, technique, alternate methods, and complications. A list of selected references for further reading is included at the end of each chapter, and some entries present viewpoints opposing those expressed in the text. With this information as a background, the student may hopefully achieve a higher level of proficiency while performing a clinical procedure than would be possible solely by the trial-and-error method.

This, then, is a book about what is commonly referred to as "scut work," a topic which continues to stimulate abundant controversy between certain academic camps. One of these feels that there is no such thing as "scut work" and that practical experience is the sine qua non of clinical training. Another, equally vehement, states that there is no time or place for the repetition of menial tasks in the student's day; his time is better spent in the library, at conferences, etc. This argument is by no means close to solution and may never be completely resolved, nor is it my purpose at this time to cast a vote with either side. I simply suggest that this book might help achieve something of a compromise. Assuming there will always be "scut work" to do, isn't it advisable to learn at an early stage of training to perform it as rapidly, efficiently, and effectively as possible? The idea for a basic guide such as this one arose during my own clinical clerkship and has been completed with just this purpose and audience in mind.

Nevertheless, despite the fact that this book is primarily oriented to the medical student, I did not lose sight of its potential usefulness to other "students of medicine" such as professional nurses, laboratory technicians, and other physician's assistants, who find themselves at one time or another in the position of performing some of the procedures discussed or else assisting the doctor with the rest. Therefore, the text dealing with technique is not encumbered with unnecessary technical jargon and does not presuppose extensive clinical experience on the part of the reader. Sections dealing with indications, interpretation, and complications naturally demand a greater understanding of the basic medical sciences.

I would like to express appreciation to the following individuals who served as my "panel of experts" and who proposed several valuable additions, corrections, and deletions: Dr. Stanley M. Goldberg, Department of Surgery, University of Minnesota Hospitals, Minneapolis; Drs. Karoly Balogh, Department of Pathology, and James L. Vanderveen, Department of Anesthesia, University Hospital, Boston; Dr. Harold W. Harrower, Department of Surgery, Veterans Administration Hospital, Providence, Rhode Island; Drs. Williams McCabe and Andrew Huvos, Department of Medicine, Boston University School of Medicine; Drs. Donald Mahler, Department of Anesthesia, and Carl Olsson, Department of Urology, Veterans Administration Hospital, Boston; Miss Emily Feener, Boston University School of Nursing; and Drs. Robert L. Berger, James A. Bougas, Richard H. Egdahl, Herbert B. Hechtman, Irving L. Madoff, John A. Mannick, and Edward L. Spatz, Department of Surgery, Boston University Medical Center.

In addition, it should be emphasized that the final content of this book is in large measure a result of the labors of numerous Boston medical students, who read the preliminary drafts and served as my severest critics. It was through their reactions, both negative and positive, that I learned exactly what they wanted to know and in what terms they understood it best.

Special thanks are to be accorded to Joan Sheahan for her lucid illustrations and to the editorial staff of Williams & Wilkins for their assistance and patience while waiting for the completion of this project.

JACK C. FISHER, M.D.

# Contents

# ONE

# Approaching the Patient

Thomas Jefferson once said, "The art of living is the art of avoiding pain." In like manner, the art of performing clinical procedures is, in large measure, the art of avoiding pain. To be sure, one also wishes to obtain the necessary specimens or desired data, but patients will judge physicians primarily by the amount of pain that they inflict. The patient does not know your academic standing or what you read the night before. He only knows that he is going to feel pain and does not like it. Some will express their fear, others will not, but all experience a variable degree of anxiety and apprehension.

Patients differ greatly according to their own personality traits as well as their recent experience. Some are almost hysterically sensitive to pain while others retain a stoic composure beyond belief. A patient who has recently taken ill may tolerate much more pain and discomfort than a chronically ill patient who has spent the last several weeks in a hospital with daily exposure to syringes, needles, and similar weapons. Therefore, it is important to know your patient well, including a little of his recent experience.

While learning to perform clinical procedures, there are a number of habits worth developing which contribute to greater patient comfort as well as diminish pain and anxiety. Speed is of the essence. Not irrational and careless speed but, rather, expeditious performance of the assigned task. All necessary equipment should be assembled before entering the patient's room since nothing is more annoying to patient and doctor alike than the necessity of making several extra trips down the hall for missing items. The nurse can be of inestimable value in this department, but she should avoid delivering the desired items too far in advance of your arrival or the patient will simply stare at the assembled gadgetry and brood about the suffering to come.

It is commonplace for doctors and nurses to announce to patients, far in advance, that a given procedure is to be carried out. Although some preparation is necessary, the time interval between the announcement and the deed should be limited. Perhaps the best time to prepare the patient verbally is when you arrive in the room to complete the task. In this way, patients will not worry for hours about what is going to happen to them.

The first thing that any patient will want to know is what is to be done, why, and will it hurt? Since there should be a good reason for every clinical procedure, there is every reason to keep the patient informed. In fact, the more that he knows about why the procedure is essential to his welfare, the more cooperative he should be.

Although some hospitals (particularly government institutions) demand written consent for each and every procedure, the request for permission should be presented to the patient in such a way that he feels he has little option to refuse. By that, I mean that it is best to be firm and authoritative, stressing that no other course is reasonable. Such an approach, if presented in a pleasant manner, will do much to gain the patient's cooperation.

Regarding the question of pain, it is never wise to merely say "No, it won't hurt at all" if it is going to. This will simply destroy the patient's confidence in you. Honesty is a better alternative. State quite frankly that "It will hurt a little, and it lasts but a few seconds." If a local anesthetic is to be used, stress this fact since knowledge that the area to be worked on will be numbed is a great reliever of anxiety.

Give some advance thought to how much pain will be involved. If it is considerable, then prescribe a sedative or an analgesic. Extensive wound debridement should always be preceded by an injection for pain. Many other procedures fall in this category as well. The drugs (e.g., barbiturates, valium, demoral, morphine) may be given intramuscularly by the nurse about 30 minutes before your arrival or else by yourself intravenously just before starting. Dosage must be adjusted according to the patient's weight and age, and great caution be exercised with the young and the aged.

The problem of judging pain is not always easy, particularly for those who have not experienced the procedure themselves. William Mayo underwent surgery early in his career and later said that it was one of his greatest learning experiences. We cannot all be on the other side of the needle or knife, but a sensitive observer should be perceptive of his patient's discomfort.

In addition to systemic sedative, analgesic and local anesthesia, a gentle and skilled hand will also prevent considerable pain. Brusque movements will merely anger the patient, regardless of how much advance medication has been given. Also recall that conversation throughout the procedure is perhaps the most effective sedative of them all.

Skillful suggestion often lessens the memory of discomfort. Upon completion of the procedure, say something like, "That didn't hurt very badly, did it?" Some will say yes, but a vast majority will admit that there was far less pain than they had anticipated and will therefore be far more receptive in case the procedure must be repeated. Patients often remember saying that the procedure did not hurt badly (even when it did).

## CHILDREN

Approaching the child can be, and usually is, a far greater challenge. Infants will usually cry regardless of your preparation and, therefore, it is wisest to proceed quickly and get the job done. Babies fortunately forget their experiences quickly, and some procedures, such as external jugular venipuncture, may be facilitated by crying.

Children from 3–16 vary in their response. Some 4 year olds will sit quietly while a sizable laceration is sutured, whereas certain 14 year olds will cry in anticipation of a simple venipuncture. You should be able to size up your patient quickly and take the appropriate measures. Some can be talked through a procedure without excessive restraint, while others must be wrapped firmly.

Nursing assistance is essential when dealing with young children. Not only can they help to control the child physically but, also, they can provide consolation while you concentrate on the assigned task. It is preferable for the baby's own parents to be out of sight and beyond hearing range while procedures are being carried out.

# THE DIFFICULT PATIENT

Despite all efforts to the contrary, there will still be a few patients who defy rational management and refuse to cooperate. Restraint is occasionally needed for the confused and irrational adult. If general obstinacy or adamant refusal prevents the completion of a procedure, notify a senior physician (preferably the patient's) rather than force the issue or waste further time.

In conclusion, if the art of performing clinical procedures lies in the avoidance of pain, then its instruments are careful preparation, firm persuasion, close attention to important details, and a gentle but quick hand. From the pen of Margaret Junkin Preston comes the apt phrase, "Pain is no longer pain when it is past." The duty of the physician performing any procedure is to make it—and the pain—past!

### Selected References for Further Reading

1. Adriani, J. Local and regional anesthesia for minor surgery. *Surg. Clin. N. Amer. 31:* 1507–1529, 1951.
2. Beecher, H. K. Pain and some factors that modify it. *Anesthesiology 12:* 633–641, 1951.
3. Bird, B. *Talking with Patients.* J. B. Lippincott, Philadelphia, 1955.
4. McKittrick, L. S. Shattuck lecture: The patient. *New Eng. J. Med. 256:* 1211–1215, 1957.

# TWO

# Venipuncture

The modern practice of medicine requires easy access to the circulatory system. The venous system being most superficial, venipuncture necessarily becomes one of the most frequently performed of all clinical procedures. Accurate laboratory diagnostic methods demand frequent collection of blood samples, and the ability to enter a vein efficiently for the purpose of administering drugs can be of lifesaving value. The removal of blood for therapeutic reasons (phlebotomy), although once practiced widely, is rarely, if ever, applied to patients with congestive heart failure in whom reduction of an expanded blood volume is of paramount need. This chapter considers all three of these applications of venipuncture and also discusses the technique of arterial puncture.

## HISTORY

Long before the circulation was adequately understood, physicians recognized a need to enter the venous system. The history of venipuncture is, therefore, intimately related to the development of phlebotomy or bloodletting as a means of therapy. Blood was recognized as "the seat of life" as well as the harbor of numerous and yet undefined diseases. Although only one of a number of "humors," it was most readily available to the medical practitioner so that the letting of blood for the purpose of eliminating disease rapidly achieved popularity.

Numerous methods of drawing blood were applied. Scarification of the skin with shells, flint stones, fish horns, and teeth was carried out in order to produce a bleeding surface. Primitive South American tribes shot small arrows into different parts of the body until a vein was pierced. The Incas of Peru refined the approach somewhat, opening a visible vein directly with sharp stones but taking particular care to locate their venesection over the site of pain, e.g. between the eyebrows in the case of headache!

Small cups were placed over scarified areas of skin in order to facilitate blood withdrawal. However, greatest reliance was placed on the use of the leech, noted for fixing itself to the skin, piercing the dermis, sucking blood until it became engorged, and then falling off. If it became necessary to remove a leech before it was satiated, salt was sprinkled on the skin and it promptly dropped off. If the leech was required to continue its function after becoming engorged, the tail was simply snipped off. Some overzealous physicians were known to apply as many as 50 leeches at one time.

Bloodletting was common practice well into the 19th century. George Washington's final illness, acute tracheobronchitis, was unsuccessfully treated by the removal of 2½ quarts of blood in a 13-hour period. By this time, however, small hollow quills were used to pierce the vein. The invention ultimately led to the practice of infusing blood and other medicaments into the circulation, a much more useful application than large scale exsanquination! From the quill, it was then only a matter of time before the appearance of fine silver tubes—and then needles as we know them today.

## EQUIPMENT

Very little is required for a simple venipuncture. Select a tourniquet (usually a short length of rubber tubing or penrose drain). The skin may be cleansed with a gauze sponge and antiseptic; e.g. povidone-iodine. Label all blood specimen tubes in advance with the patient's name. After determining the volume of blood required, select a syringe of appropriate size. An 18- or 20-gauge needle is ideal for collecting blood samples. Smaller needles (e.g. 22- or 25-gauge) may produce slightly less discomfort but the syringe will fill too slowly and the blood may either hemolyze or clot. Larger needles (17- or 14-gauge) require local anesthesia before use and are unnecessary for blood collection. Whenever drugs are administered intravenously, either fill the syringe yourself or accept it only from the nurse who filled it (who should state the dose contained within and allow you to read the label on the container).

## NEEDED FOR VENIPUNCTURE:

Tourniquet (short length of rubber tubing)
Prep sponge and antiseptic
Syringe or Vacutainer

18- or 20-gauge needle
Specimen tubes (prelabeled)
Band-Aid (optional)

## TECHNIQUE

Patients should be sitting or lying but *never* standing. The robust individual who "can take it standing" is the most likely to fall! Apply a tourniquet promptly to the upper arm to allow for venous distention while syringe, needle, etc., are being readied. With the patient opening and closing his hand in a fist formation, the veins soon dilate. Patients dislike this procedure so that it is wise to work quickly at this point without displaying the needle prominently.

The most common site selected for draining blood samples is the antecubital fossa (Fig. 2.1). The basilic, cephalic, and median cubital veins are ordinarily large and close to the surface here, but the median antibrachial or accessory cephalic at the wrist are also suitable.

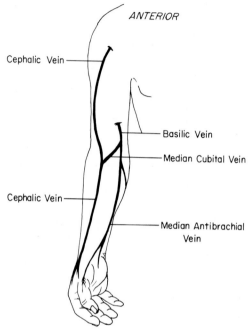

**Figure 2.1.** Superficial veins of the arm.

Grasp the arm firmly with one hand so that the thumb holds the skin taut just distal to the venipuncture site (Fig. 2.2). Cleanse the skin with a cotton pledget held in the other hand. Do not discard the pledget but rather set it nearby, preferably on its sterile wrapper, and pick up the previously prepared syringe and needle. Insert the needle in two steps. First, with the bevel of the needle up, pierce the skin just to the side of the vein. Once through the skin, reassure the patient and say that the greatest discomfort is over. Now change the direction of the needle slightly, aim it toward the side of the vein while applying slight back pressure on the syringe plunger, and advance slowly. Entrance of the vein should be heralded by the return of blood. If, on the other hand, both the skin and vein are pierced with one thrust, there is far greater chance of

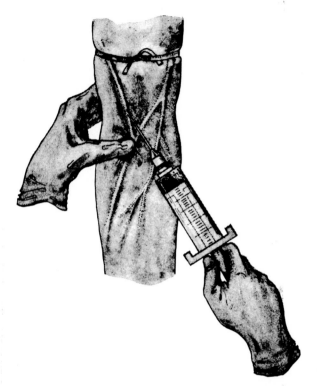

**Figure 2.2.** Grasp the arm firmly with one hand so that the thumb holds the skin taut just distal to the intended venipuncture site.

failure, since patients often jump—resulting in either a complete miss or else puncture of both the anterior and posterior walls of the vein. There is also quicker sealing and less bleeding if the side of the vein is entered. After withdrawing sufficient blood, release the tourniquet, place the nearby pledget over the puncture site, and remove the needle. If the patient is cooperative, ask him to raise his arm and hold pressure over the gauze pad. If the patient is not able to help, than an assistant will be necessary to exert pressure on the wound while you distribute the blood specimen among the prepared tubes. Particular care must be devoted to preserving the integrity of the vein because you are quite likely to be back another day and therefore do not wish a hematoma to develop. If many tubes of blood are required, a Vacutainer can be used (Fig. 2.3).

When administering medications by vein, the same procedure is followed except that, after entering the vein, the tourniquet is released immediately, 1–2 cc of blood are aspirated to ensure proper positioning of the needle, and the drug is injected slowly. If there is any doubt about the needle's position, or if injection evokes pain, or if there are signs of local swelling, then extravasation of drug has occurred and the procedure should be terminated at once! Attempts at this point to reposition the needle are rarely successful without further infiltration of drug into the surrounding tissue. Remember to accept drugs only from the nurse who filled the syringe. She should restate the dosage and display the drug label to you as well.

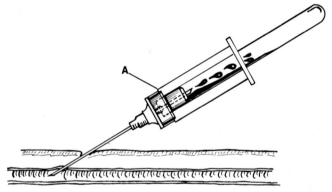

**Figure 2.3.** The Vacutainer method of venipuncture. A collection tube is placed into the Vacutainer and advanced to the line (A). The needle is then inserted into a vein using the techniques similar to those described for venipuncture with a syringe. The collection tube is advanced onto the needle in the Vacutainer. When the needle is inside the vein, blood will flow into the vacuum of the collection tube. Holding the Vacutainer assembly steady, multiple tubes may be placed into the chamber to remove blood for various reasons.

## SPECIAL PROBLEMS

### Infants

With the development of microtechniques in the laboratory, smaller volumes of venous blood are now required. Simple heel puncture will often be sufficient to obtain blood in capillary tubes. This is fortunate, since extracting blood from the veins of infants can be a trying experience.

The external jugular vein is a frequently used site, although prominent veins in the arm and hand may also be punctured if they are apparent. On the other hand, it is often difficult to find veins on the limbs and, when present, it is wiser to save them for intravenous infusions. The femoral vein should be avoided in children because of the frequency of complications attending its use. This is discussed later. Ask the nurse to wrap the child in a sheet and hold the head to one side. Crying and straining are almost inevitable but they usually serve to make the vein more prominent. Steady the vein proximally and distally with two fingers and puncture the vein in the line of blood flow, i.e. aiming toward the thorax.

### The Elderly

Venipuncture can be most difficult in the elderly, even when their veins are prominent. Choosing a less prominent vein, i.e. one set within the subcutaneous tissue, is wiser than selecting the boldest vessel in view which is likely to roll easily, is hard to immobilize, and frequently shatters when punctured. A very steady hand and intense concentration are required in this situation. Also, pressure must be applied for 4–5 minutes after venipuncture in order to prevent a hematoma.

### "No Veins"

Venipuncture can be the easiest of techniques and also the most trying, particularly in the patient whose veins are inaccessible because of obesity or repeated venipunctures during a prolonged hospitalization. When having difficulty, there are a number of precautions which may be taken. First, switch from a simple tourniquet (which achieves only 30–40 mm of pressure—more will be too painful) to a blood pressure cuff inflated nearly to the diastolic arterial pressure. Theoretically, the veins should be maximally distended with a tourniquet but this does not hold true in practice. Blood pressure cuffs often bring out veins which are not apparent with a tourniquet. Warm packs may also promote venous dilation.

In the event of repeated failure, it is more merciful to perform a rapid, efficient femoral vein puncture than to cause the patient persistent pain in the pursuit of a peripheral vein.

### Femoral Vein Puncture

This procedure is quite easy to perform with very little discomfort to the patient. While standing on the same side as the vein to be tapped, abduct the leg slightly and palpate the femoral artery just inferior to the inguinal ligament. With fingers of one hand still in place over the point of maximal pulsation, cleanse the skin just medial to the fingertips, set the gauze pledget nearby, insert the needle 0.5–1.0 cm medial to your fingertips, and advance downward slowly while applying constant back pressure on the syringe plunger (Fig. 2.4B). If blood is not encountered, withdraw the tip of the needle almost to the level of the skin before changing direction slightly or else the tip may injure the vessel. After withdrawing sufficient blood, apply pressure over the vein for 2–3 minutes.

### Femoral Artery Puncture

It is often necessary to obtain arterial blood for pH and blood gas determination. The two sites most commonly used are the radial and femoral arteries. The latter is easiest to puncture.

Standing on the side of patient *opposite* to the artery to be tapped, abduct the leg and palpate the artery. Now follow the same procedure as with vein tap except that the needle should pierce the skin lateral to the fingertips (Fig. 2.4A). Pull the skin slightly in the medial direction and the needle should come to

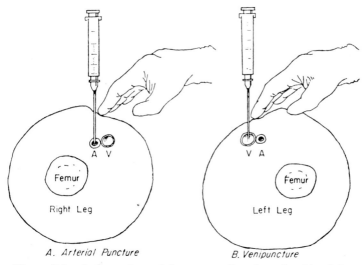

A. Arterial Puncture

B. Venipuncture

**Figure 2.4.** A, femoral arterial puncture. Stand on the side of the patient opposite to the leg used and insert the needle slightly lateral to the point of maximum pulsation. B, femoral vein puncture. Stand on the same side as the vein to be tapped and insert the needle slightly medial to the point of maximum pulsation.

the artery first. Check this by noting the color of the blood or, if necessary, remove the syringe from the needle briefly to detect pulsation. Radiologists performing arteriograms, who must be certain that their needles are well placed, wear gloves and always check by removing the syringe and adjusting the needle until vigorous pulsations are seen. After aspiration of blood, firm pressure (5–6 minutes) is mandatory or hematomas will commonly develop.

### Radial Artery Puncture

The radial artery has become a popular vessel for obtaining arterial blood. The two major advantages of the radial artery are its superficial location and its lack of an accompanying vein. Any blood drawn will usually be arterial blood.

The radial pulse is familiar to everyone as the time-honored place where the "heart" rate is measured. It is medial to the radial styloid at the distal end of the radius. The skin is prepared with povidone-iodine and the artery is located about 1 cm proximal to the tip of the radial styloid. The needle (25-gauge, ⅝-inch) is introduced perpendicular to the skin over the artery and the artery impaled with the needle (Fig. 2.5). If the needle is advanced too far, it should be withdrawn a sufficient distance to allow free flow of blood into the syringe. After removing the needle, keep pressure on the site for 5–6 minutes (by the clock). All arterial blood for blood gas determination should be heparinized and promptly transported on ice to the laboratory.

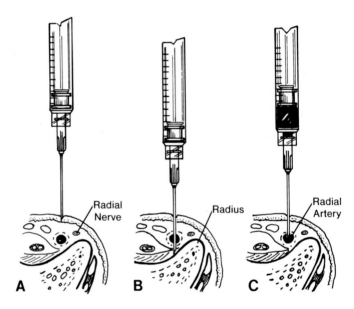

**Figure 2.5.** Radial artery puncture. The radial artery is impaled with a needle (B) and withdrawn until there is a free flow of blood into the syringe (C).

# COMPLICATIONS

The very careless and sometimes the very careful physician will produce a hematoma at the site of the venipuncture. This in itself is no serious problem except that the vein is then rendered useless for either blood collection or intravenous infusions for several days or weeks. More serious, however, is the infiltration of drugs into the tissues around the vein. Some drugs may occasionally produce skin necrosis if extravasion is extensive, norepinephrine being the best example. In the event of norepinephrine infiltration, infiltration of an adrenergic blocking agent such as Regitine becomes necessary. Bromsulphalein dye and Adriamycin can also be painful and result in skin necrosis.

Phlebitis is a rare complication of simple venipuncture, and is more often associated with long-term placement of needles or catheters within veins. However, the single injection of some cancer chemotherapeutic drugs (e.g. 5-FUDR) may incite an acute phlebitic reaction.

Femoral taps are ordinarily safe in adults but are dangerous in infants for at least two reasons. First, the joint space of the hip is easily entered if the needle is advanced too far, and osteomyelitis stemming from such a procedure is periodically reported. Second, the threat of vascular injury exists. Isolated reports of gangrenous extremities resulting from simple femoral vein puncture are sufficient reason to avoid this site in young children.

Femoral artery sticks may also be dangerous in the elderly since the procedure may dislodge arteriosclerotic plaques. Such vascular injuries can induce embolization or thrombosis, either of which could result in loss of part or all of the lower extremity.

## Selected References for Further Reading

1. Adriani, J. Venipuncture. *Amer. J. Nursing 62:* 66–70, 1962.
2. Centerwall, W. R. The venipuncture in pediatrics. *GP 15:* 74–79, 1957.
3. Clark, R. B. The art of venipuncture. *New Physician 13:* 253–256, 1964.
4. Nabseth, D. C. and Jones, J. E. Gangrene of the lower extremities of infants after femoral venipuncture. *New Eng. J. Med. 268:* 1003–1005, 1963.

# THREE

# Intravenous Infusions

Starting an intravenous infusion involves little more than a standard venipuncture, plus a few precautions to ensure that the needle (or catheter) remains in place for a useful period of time. Most important among these precautions are the selection of the right vein, insertion of the most appropriate cannula, and application of sufficient restraint to prevent dislodgement or fluid infiltration. Each of these is discussed in detail together with several basic principles of intravenous infusion therapy.

## HISTORY

The development of modern parenteral fluid therapy probably began in 1665 when Sir Christopher Wren, a professional architect and amateur physiologist, first fashioned primitive needles from feather quills. Working with two associates, Robert Boyle and John Wilkins, he injected wine, ale, opium, and numerous other substances into the veins of dogs. This occurred at a time when the practice of phlebotomy was widespread, and out of this experience Wren developed the idea that stimulants or "good blood" might be reinfused into those patients from whom "evil blood" had been taken.

There were many scattered reports of blood transfusion in man during the 17th and 18th centuries. However, most of these are difficult to substantiate because it was common practice at the time for warriors to drink the blood of their enemies following military victory in order to regain vigor for future battles. Therefore, many of these early reports actually involved "oral blood transfusion." One typical example was the unsuccessful attempt to prolong the life of Pope Innocent VIII with infants' blood.

One early case of human blood transfusion is more than adequately documented as a result of the legal battle which followed. Beginning in 1667, Richard Lower of Oxford gave sheep's blood to several patients with infrequent success. One patient was given multiple transfusions and died of anaphylaxis after the third administration. The patient's widow promptly instituted court proceedings, which resulted in a law forbidding all subsequent transfusion of blood in Great Britain.

Successful blood replacement did not again take place until the beginning of the 20th century when Landsteiner defined the major blood groups. The practice of intravenous fluid therapy appeared several decades later when a better understanding of the dynamics of body fluid physiology developed.

## EQUIPMENT

Fortunately, feather quills have lost their popularity, and even the stainless steel needle now appears to be destined for extinction. During the past several years, numerous disposable percutaneous needle-catheter units have become available which permit cannulation of veins without surgical exposure.

Whether one uses a simple needle or a catheter depends on several factors. If the patient requires a single infusion, or if maintenance fluids are to be administered in 3–6 hours and then discontinued, a needle will be perfectly adequate. However, if the patient is in need of rapid blood volume replacement, is destined for the operating room, or requires total fluid maintenance for several days, then it is wise to insert a plastic catheter into a large vein. Percutaneous needle-catheter units such as the Angiocath involve a beveled cannula which surrounds a smaller needle.

Parenteral fluids may be administered through a 22-gauge

needle, but blood and other colloids flow better through an 18- or 19-gauge needle. (Remember that needles increase in diameter as their numbers decrease.) Rapid blood replacement requires at least a 17-gauge needle or catheter. Infants may be given small volumes of blood through a 21-gauge needle, but sludging will take place following prolonged administration through anything less than a 19-gauge needle. Scalp vein needles are specially designed for the small delicate veins found in infants, and can be quite useful in adults (Fig. 3.1).

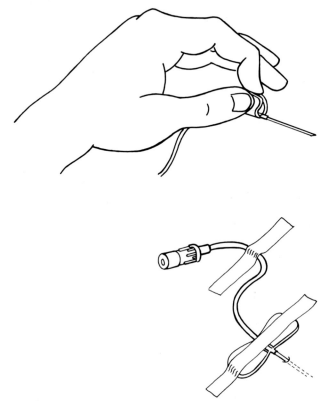

**Figure 3.1.** Scalp vein needle insertion can be accomplished by using the wings to control the insertion.

In addition to the prescribed fluid, the minimum equipment for starting an intravenous infusion are a prep sponge, an intravenous tubing set, a needle, and adhesive tape. If a large caliber needle (greater than 18-gauge) is to be inserted, anesthetize the skin with 1% Lidocaine before starting. If a plastic catheter is to be inserted for several days, use additional sterility precautions; i.e. povidone-iodine skin prep beforehand and antibiotic ointment afterward.

---

## NEEDED FOR STARTING AN INTRAVENOUS INFUSION:

Tourniquet

Intravenous fluid (prelabeled)

Intravenous tubing set

Appropriate cannula (e.g. needle, Angiocath, scalp vein set, etc.)

Prep sponge and antiseptic

Local anesthetic (optional)

Antibiotic ointment

Adhesive tape

Armboard (optional)

---

## SITE SELECTION

The upper extremity should be the first choice for intravenous infusions. Avoid the lower extremity because of the risk of thrombophlebitis. Select a fairly straight vein so that the needle can be advanced into the lumen for a distance of 1–2 cm. Needles should never be placed in veins where they cross a joint, e.g. the wrist or antecubital fossa, since sudden arm movement may result in a torn vein and fluid infiltration. Only flexible catheters may be placed safely in the large veins at the elbow. Veins on the dorsum of the hand are not satisfactory when drugs are to be administered, for if infiltration does occur, there is an increased chance of injury to the skin. Use the forearm instead.

In the absence of suitable arm veins, the external jugular

vein may be cannulated percutaneously with a catheter. Otherwise, a vein must be exposed surgically (cutdown). The leg should not be used except for emergencies such as cardiac arrest, when a rapid temporary cutdown can be performed using the greater saphenous vein at the groin or ankle.

## TECHNIQUE

First, apply a tourniquet and ask the patient to open and close his fist several times in order to produce venous distention. While waiting a few moments, connect the infusion set, hang the bottle of fluid on an overhead stand, and fill the drip chamber and tubing. Recap the needle tip and set it nearby. Select a suitable vein and cleanse the skin with antiseptic.

When using a needle, proceed as you would for any venipuncture. If the vein is deep or appears difficult to puncture, it is wise to use a syringe so that the correct positioning of the needle within the lumen can be confirmed by withdrawing a small volume of blood. Prominent veins ordinarily can be punctured directly, with the needle already connected to the IV tubing. With experience, you will be able to feel the tip enter the vein, but its position can be checked best by squeezing the rubber bulb near the needle hub, looking for blood return. Advance the needle 1–2 cm into the lumen, check its position again, remove the tourniquet, and begin the infusion slowly. Watch for local induration, which, if present, indicates incorrect needle placement. If the skin over the tip appears normal and the drip rate is adequate, finish by adequately taping the needle in place. Small armboards are also helpful for immobilization (Fig. 3.2).

When inserting an Angiocath or similar needle/catheter unit, attach a syringe and advance the needle tip into a vein as described above. Make certain that the lumen has been entered by aspirating a small volume of blood. Then, simultaneously advance the outer catheter and withdraw the inner needle, and finish by connecting the intravenous line and starting the infusion (Fig. 3.3).

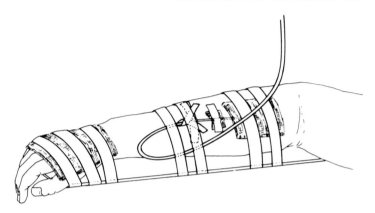

**Figure 3.2.** The use of an armboard and wisely placed adhesive tape immobilizes the needle and prevents infiltration.

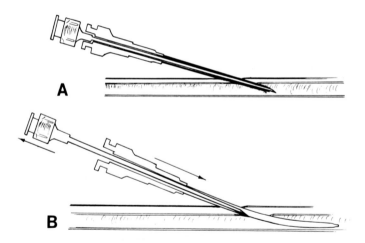

**Figure 3.3.** Insertion of angiocath. A, perform venipuncture. B, simultaneously advance outer catheter and withdraw inner needle.

Whenever plastic catheters are inserted, prep the skin extremely well in advance and apply antibiotic ointment afterward. Change the dressings over indwelling catheters every 2 days.

## MAINTENANCE

Malfunction of an intravenous infusion is usually related to catheter and needle movement. Therefore, attention to proper restraint is mandatory. Flexible catheters tolerate a small amount of movement, but needles tolerate none at all! A slow infusion rate may be due either to sludging of blood within the lumen, or else to angulation of the needle so that the bevel rests against the wall of the vein. Irrigation with 10 cc of sterile saline usually solves the first problem and additional adhesive tape ordinarily counteracts the second.

In order to prevent clotting of catheters which are to be left in place several days, place 1000–2000 USP units of heparin in each liter of fluid. The systemic clotting time will not be affected, but local thrombosis within the catheter lumen is effectively diminished.

## RATES OF INFUSION

No sensible physician would leave an order for morphine or digitalis without specifying the dose and frequency of administration. Parenteral fluid therapy deserves as much consideration as any drug, since underinfusion can lead to dehydration or electrolyte imbalance, and overinfusion might result in cardiac decompensation. All fluid orders must, therefore, include specific instructions as to total volume as well as infusion speed.

In order to define maximum infusion limits, consider the condition of the patient as well as the composition of the fluid. Is the patient a young child or a fully grown adult? Is he already dehydrated or in reasonable fluid balance? Is he a cardiac cripple on digitalis or in excellent cardiovascular health? What volume of fluid is to be administered and does it contain potassium, glucose, sodium, or colloid? All of these factors must be evaluated before determining infusion rates.

The healthy adult can receive 500 ml of fluid/hour safely, but elderly patients or those with cardiac disease should receive no more than 300 ml/hour, and even less if the solution contains sodium. Therefore, 3000 ml may be given in 6–9 hours depending on the patient's status. Severely dehydrated patients may receive much higher rates of infusion. If losses and maintenance fluids are infused over a 24-hour period, then slower rates, e.g. 100–200 ml/hour, are more appropriate.

Excessive glucose infusion may present too great an osmotic load to the kidney, resulting in diuresis and, ultimately, dehydration. The normal adult should receive no more than 0.5 to 0.6 g/kg/hour of glucose. In a 60-kg patient, this represents 360 ml/hour of 10% glucose or 720 ml/hour of 5% glucose. Starved dehydrated patients should receive no more than 0.5 g/kg/hour (i.e. 180 ml of 10% glucose/hour or 360 ml of 5% glucose/hour).

Rates of potassium infusion should be limited to 20 mEq/hour. No more than 40–60 mEq of potassium chloride should be added to each liter of fluid unless it is infused very slowly, since higher concentrations at normal rates will produce muscle spasm and local pain.

Colloidal solutions are usually administered more slowly than crystalloids unless they are being given to expand a depleted blood volume. A patient in hypovolemic shock needs blood as fast as it can be infused, whereas a cardiac patient should not be given more than 250 ml of packed red cells in a 2-hour period. Severely chronically anemic patients should receive blood at even slower rates, since their blood volumes are already expanded maximally.

Fluid rates in children must be calculated according to weight, or even better, according to body surface area. Maintenance fluid therapy ranges from 1200 to 1500 ml/m$^2$/day, but excessive losses may call for higher infusion rates.

Do not attach a 1000-ml bottle of fluid into a small infant's intravenous line since inadvertent rapid infusion could lead to tragic consequences. Rather, parenteral fluids in children should be delivered via 250 and 500 ml bottles and through a 100-ml Volutrol.

## COMPLICATIONS

1. Infiltration represents not only the most frequent complication of intravenous infusion, but also one of the greatest sources of annoyance and wasted time for medical students, house officers, and nurses alike. Although some elderly patients have veins which are so fragile that they defy even the lowest infusion pressure, most of the time infiltration of fluid into the subcutaneous tissue is a result of excess needle movement and laceration of the vein wall. Therefore, infiltration can usually be prevented by careful fixation of the needle with sufficient adhesive tape. Restive patients must be restrained *before* they dislodge or pull out their intravenous infusion, not afterward. Members of the family often become alarmed at the sight of arm restraints so they should be told that the drugs received by vein are absolutely essential, and that the discomfort associated with repeated venipunctures is far greater than that experienced from arm restraint.

The best way to determine whether infiltration has occurred is to feel the skin over the needle. If it is swollen and cold and the needle tip cannot be felt, then the infusion must be re-established in another vein. The zone of infiltration usually recedes in 24 hours, or faster, if warm packs are applied. However, if the infusion contains a powerful vasoconstrictor, such as Levophed, then there is danger of skin necrosis, and the area must be infiltrated with an adrenergic blocking agent such as Regitine (10 mg diluted in 20 ml of saline).

2. Phlebitis or chemical inflammation caused by plastic cannulas in the upper extremity is not uncommon, and can be recognized by the development of local pain, swelling, and erythema, often extending to the shoulder. The most common time for this to occur is after 72 hours (i.e. "third day fever").

Embolism is quite unusual, however. Treatment consists of prompt removal of the offending cannula and application of warm packs. Fonkalsrud has called attention to the acidity of dextrose solutions (pH 3–5) as one cause of phlebitis and advocates buffering these fluids with sodium bicarbonate (0.6–0.7 g or 7–9 mEq/liter).

3. Septicemia associated with long-term catheter placement is a rapidly increasing clinical problem. A study by Bentley and Lepper demonstrated that almost half of the hospital-acquired septicemias are now a result of in-dwelling catheters. The reported septicemia rate for 756 patients with catheters in place for 48 hours was 2.5%. This is a serious problem and one which requires preventive measures. Among these are 1) a very careful skin prep, 2) aseptic technique, 3) application of anti-biotic ointment at the catheter site, 4) dressing change, re-application of antibiotic ointment, and close inspection of the site for evidence of phlebitis or infection every 2 days, and 5) removal of all catheters at the first sign of local inflammation or unexplained sepsis. Also remember to culture the catheter tip!

4. Embolization of pieces of plastic catheters became wide-spread shortly after the introduction of percutaneous needle-catheter units. Catheters might migrate to the right heart if they are cut at skin level with the sharp point of an Intracath needle. Treatment of this unfortunate complication may re-quire open heart surgery and can be prevented by remembering to slide the protective plastic shield over the point of the needle where the catheter emerges. Also, secure both needle and catheter to a tongue blade with adhesive tape. Careful taping of the plastic cannula to the skin eliminates the chance of embolization following accidental transection of the catheter.

### Selected References for Further Reading

1. Bentley, D. W. and Lepper, M. H. Septicemia related to indwelling venous catheter. *J.A.M.A. 206:* 1749–1752, 1968.
2. Fonkalsrud, E. W., Pederson, D. M., Murphy, J., and Beckerman, J. H. Reduction of infusion thrombophlebitis with buffered glucose solutions. *Surgery 63:* 280–284, 1968.

3. Knight, R. J. Flow rates through disposable intravenous cannulae. *Lancet* 2: 665–667, 1968.
4. McCabe, W. R. and Jackson, G. G. Gram-negative bacteremia: etiology and ecology. *Arch. Intern. Med. (Chicago) 110:* 847–855, 1962.
5. *Parenteral Administration.* Abbott Laboratories, Chicago, 1959.
6. Tarail, R. Practice of fluid therapy. *J.A.M.A. 171:* 45–49, 1959.
7. Wilmore, D. W. and Dudrick, S. J. Safe long-term venous catheterization. *Arch. Surg. (Chicago) 98:* 256–258, 1969.

# FOUR

# The Cutdown

Despite the very best efforts of an experienced hand, there are certain clinical situations when an intravenous infusion cannot be started with a needle. The patient may be in shock with no venous distention, or obesity and chronic hospitalization may have obscured all available veins. In these instances, surgical exposure of a vein, or cutdown, becomes necessary. The procedure is quite simple and is usually far less time-consuming than an endless futile search for small veins which will not admit a needle successfully. In addition, cutting down on a peripheral vein is the procedure of choice for rapid access to the circulation in the event of cardiac arrest.

Some house officers never become proficient at cutdowns and a few actively avoid doing them. This unnecessary fear of the procedure is probably derived from two specific problems, namely, locating a suitable vein and getting the catheter into the lumen. This chapter discusses general cutdown technique and specifically describes how to solve these two problems.

## SITE SELECTION

In the event of circulatory failure of any cause, venous distention rapidly disappears and percutaneous needle insertion becomes virtually impossible. In this case, the greater saphenous vein should be exposed at the ankle (1 cm anterior and 1 cm proximal to the medial malleolus) as quickly as possible and a large bore catheter inserted. *In all other situations, the ankle should be avoided because of the frequent association of phlebitis with lower extremity indwelling catheters.*

The upper arm is the most frequently used site for a cutdown. The cephalic vein lies superficial to the musculature just lateral to the body of the biceps brachialis. It is rarely thrombosed, even after numerous intravenous infusions have been started in the lower arm. The antecubital fossa is ordinarily a poor site since all accessible veins have usually been used for venipuncture, and the incidence of thrombosis and perivascular hematoma is high. A vein in the lower arm which cannot be cannulated percutaneously is suitable for cutdowns, but make certain that it is soft since frequently utilized veins in the lower arm are often thrombosed.

If the cephalic vein has already been used in the mid-upper arm, it can be entered at the shoulder where it passes through the deltopectoral groove. The dissection may need to be extended into the muscle tissue since the vein frequently lies hidden between the borders of the two muscles. The external jugular vein is also an excellent cutdown site, particularly since a catheter in this site can serve the important function of monitoring central venous pressure.

Exposure of a vein should not be a problem if some time is devoted in advance of the incision to palpation of a suitable target. Apply a tourniquet or blood pressure cuff and look for the vein first rather than proceeding immediately in an area where a vein is supposed to lie. Lengthy "veinless" dissections in obese arms can be avoided (but not completely eliminated, unfortunately) by a little planning and forethought. However, in the best of hands, a certain number of cutdown incisions will have to be closed because of the absence of or inadequate caliber of vein. Another site should be sought. If an unsuitable or thrombosed vein is located in one arm, don't go to the same site in the other arm where the anatomy may be similar, but try rather for the external jugular vein which is more constant and easier to find.

## EQUIPMENT

Hospitals usually provide a basic tray of instruments known commonly as the "cutdown set." However, the quality of the instruments in these sets often leaves much to be desired. This is not only a result of constant instrument abuse, but also relates to the common habit of populating the trays with operating room discards. Most notably deficient is a pair of "delicate" scissors so necessary for incising the wall of the vein. Check the scissors provided and, if they appear to cut poorly, ask for a No. 11 Bard Parker scalpel blade.

Another common failing of many cutdown sets is the only silk suture is provided. This is partially explained by the fact that catgut cannot be autoclaved. However, since cutdown sites are prone to infection, silk extrusion may occur months afterward. Therefore, it is wise to ask for fine catgut (all surgical wards should stock packets of 3-0 or 4-0 plain gut) and use this to secure the cannula within the vein. Use nylon or silk only for skin closure!

Use either fine polyethylene tubing (Clay Adams, Intramedic) attached to blunt needles (size 15–18) or else select a large intracath (C. R. Bard, No. 14), dismantle it, throw the needle away, and use only the catheter. Also, be sure to ask for a decent portable spotlight since operating in the dark is seldom an enjoyable experience.

---

## NEEDED FOR A CUTDOWN:

Light

Tourniquet

Cutdown instrument set

Intravenous fluid

Intravenous tubing set

Prep sponge and antiseptic

Local anesthetic (1% Lidocaine)

Polyethylene catheter

No. 10 and 11 scalpel blades

3-0 or 4-0 catgut suture for ties
5-0 nylon suture for skin closure
Antibiotic ointment

Tongue blade
Adhesive tape
Armboard (optional)

---

## TECHNIQUE

First hang the fluid, fill the tubing, and place the tip somewhere adjacent to the planned operative field. Apply a tourniquet or blood pressure cuff and try to palpate a suitable vein. After selecting a site, maintain venous distention by keeping the tourniquet in place. Open the instrument tray, apply sterile gloves, and prep the skin widely with an appropriate antiseptic (e.g. povidone-iodine, tincture of Zephiran, etc.). Infiltrate the skin with 1% Lidocaine in a transverse line over a 3-cm length extending 1.5 cm to either side of the place where the vein is either palpated or expected to lie. By doing this, the skin will already be anesthetized if the incision needs to be extended.

At this point, prepare the cannula. Unless the catheter is tapered, cut a slight bevel in the tip to facilitate insertion. Also snip the small point off the tip of the bevel, fashioning it into a gentle curve in order to avoid piercing or injuring the intima of the vein. Finally, fill the catheter with saline.

After waiting a few moments, start with a small (1½–2 cm) transverse incision. Be sure to incise the skin completely before attempting to dissect out the vein! Many are fearful of dividing skin in one bold stroke lest they inadvertently and prematurely cut the vein. This is actually difficult to do for even though the vein appears to be 1–2 mm beneath the skin surface, it is actually far deeper. Considerable subcutaneous and perivascular connective tissue ordinarily surrounds the vein. The skin is completely incised only after the wound edges part and fatty tissue begins to protrude.

After completing the incision, lay the knife down, take a small curved hemostatic clamp, and expose the vein by using gentle spreading motions parallel to the direction of the vein.

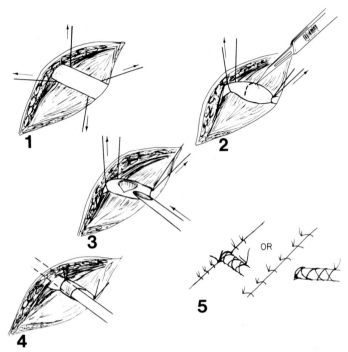

**Figure 4.1.** 1, incise the skin, expose the vein, and place two ties underneath. 2, tie the vein distally, retract with the proximal tie, and hemisect the vein. 3, carefully insert a beveled polyethylene catheter. 4, secure the catheter with the proximal tie. 5, close wound, tying catheter in place with ends of center skin suture.

As the subcutaneous layer separates, watch closely for a blue tubular structure, usually lying within the fat. Occasionally, the vein lies deep to the fat directly over muscle, in which case there may be a problem differentiating the two tissues, particularly in the absence of good lighting.

After the vessel is exposed, continue to free the lateral and inferior surfaces of their connective tissue attachments. Pass the tip of a hemostat under the vein, grasp the end of an 8-

inch length of catgut and pull it back through. Tie the vessel distally in order to occlude venous flow. Now pull a second tie under the vein in a similar fashion and grasp both ends with a hemostat. This will not be tied until after the catheter is in place, but in the meantime, it serves nicely as a vein retractor and prevents back bleeding after the vein is opened.

In order to avoid difficulty while introducing the catheter into the lumen, it is extremely important to make a precise cut in the vein wall. Hemisection seems to be ideal since a smaller hole will not admit the catheter with ease and a larger cut may soon lead to a completely divided vein. A small pointed No. 11 blade is the ideal instrument for this step. After distending the vein with blood and while maintaining tension with the proximal tie, hold the blade by the side of the vein with the cutting edge up. Starting with the tip at the "equator," advancement of the blade through the vein should result in exact hemisection.

Now lay the scalpel down and pick up the tip of the catheter. Place the beveled tip into the opening, gradually releasing tension on the proximal suture as the catheter is advanced into the lumen. Remember at this point to ask an assistant to reach under the drapes and release the tourniquet so that the catheter may be advanced easily 6–10 cm into the vein. Next, tie the proximal suture firmly enough to hold the catheter in place, but not so tight as to occlude the lumen (Fig. 4.2). A second proximal tie is often a worthwhile addition.

Connect the catheter to the nearby intravenous line immediately. If this is not done, the cannula may clot or inadvert-

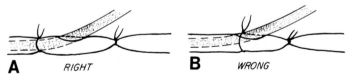

**A** RIGHT    **B** WRONG

**Figure 4.2.** A, right-vein wall must be interposed between the catheter and tie. The latter should be tight enough but yet not occlude the lumen. B, wrong—an incorrectly placed or loosely secured tie results in leakage.

ently become dislodged. The wound should then be irrigated with saline and closed with interrupted nylon sutures, one of which (usually the middle one) serves to hold the catheter in place. Apply antibiotic ointment over the incision and catheter before covering the area with a sterile dressing. This dressing and the ointment should be replaced every 2 days until the catheter is removed.

Primary healing of the cutdown incision may be facilitated and scar formation minimized by passing the catheter through a nearby but separate wound. In order to do this easily, make a small stab wound (with the No. 11 blade) 1–2 cm distal to the incision and pass the catheter tip through it before cannulating the vein. Write a note in the chart (and sometimes on the dressing if the patient is being transferred) indicating the size and length of the catheter, as well as the date and time of insertion.

## COMPLICATIONS

### Failure

There are two main reasons for failure. First is the inability to find a suitable vein, and second is the inability to insert the catheter into the lumen. The first may be kept to a minimum by looking carefully before making the incision. However, if an exposed vein is obviously too small, or filled with clot, close the wound rapidly and go on to another site rather than waste 30–60 minutes more and be left with an inadequate intravenous line. The second cause of failure is usually a result of rough handling and clumsy technique, particularly while incising the vein. If a ragged cut is made in the adventitia which misses the intima, then the catheter will simply dissect a space between the two layers and never even enter the lumen. Therefore, be sure to hemitransect the vein and look either for blood or a glistening intima. Remember, however, that all veins do not back bleed—particularly if a valve lies nearby or if the patient is in profound shock.

## Infection

The problem of local and systemic infection emanating from intravenous catheters has already been discussed under intravenous infusions. The problem applies in equal if not greater degree to cutdown since 1) they are the securest form of intravenous infusion and, unless purposely removed, will usually last the longest period of time, and 2) they are often placed hastily under less than ideal conditions, and are, as a result, more susceptible to bacterial contamination. Therefore, keep track of the length of time that a catheter is in place and remove it as soon as possible. If necessary, replace cutdowns every 4–5 days. In the presence of sepsis without obvious etiology, change all indwelling catheters and remember to culture their tips. Milk the vein back toward the opening to be sure there is no septic phlebitis.

## Phlebitis

Deep vein phlebitis and embolization from catheters in the arm are extremely rare. Chemical phlebitis, however, is not uncommon. Any sign of superficial cellulitis or pain calls for prompt removal of the offending catheter.

Superficial phlebitis in the legs associated with ankle cutdowns is far more frequent and may lead to deep vein thrombosis and pulmonary embolization. Therefore, the greater saphenous vein in the ankle should be used only for emergencies. As soon as circulation has been restored and a satisfactory vein has been cannulated in the arm or neck, promptly remove the ankle cutdown.

## Embolus

Catheter emboli are rare with cutdowns since they are ordinarily tied in place. However, overzealous tying of the catheter can lead to a retained fragment at the time of cutdown removal which then may travel proximally toward the heart. Therefore, never use force! If the catheter will not come out easily, the wound may have to be partially opened and the suture cut. The need for this is, fortunately, uncommon.

## Selected References for Further Reading

1. Indar, R. The dangers of indwelling polyethylene cannulae in deep veins. *Lancet 1:* 284–286, 1959.
2. Randolph, J. Technique for insertion of plastic catheter into saphenous vein. *Pediatrics 24:* 631–635, 1959.
3. Van Way, C. W., III. *Intravenous Techniques in Surgical Skills in Patient Care.* C. V. Mosby Company, St. Louis, 1978.

# FIVE

# Central Venous and Pulmonary Artery Catheterization

## CENTRAL VENOUS CATHETERIZATION AND CENTRAL VENOUS PRESSURE

The three indications for central venous catheterization are: central venous pressure measurement (CVP), total parenteral nutrition, and unavailability of other venous access sites. This section deals with the techniques for securing a central venous access and obtaining a CVP.

### History

Since its clinical introduction by Aubiniac in 1952, the measurement of CVP has not only achieved great popularity but also taken its well-deserved place beside more traditional means of monitoring critically ill patients, such as pulse, blood pressure, and urine output. This advance has been due, in large measure, to clinical experience and experimental evidence that has established the superiority of CVP over peripheral venous pressure as an indicator of cardiac function.

Nevertheless, central venous pressure continues to stimulate criticism perhaps because so many physicians have grown to depend too heavily on its values. Like any other clinical measurement, CVP is susceptible to errors of interpretation and may provide the unwitting physician with misleading advice. It is important to remember that the central venous pressure is not directly related to blood volume, but merely measures right ventricular end diastolic pressure, thus reflecting empirically left ventricular function. The CVP indicates how well the heart accepts and then expels the venous blood which returns to it, and therefore serves as an extremely useful guide for blood and fluid replacement.

### Site Selection

There are three suitable sites for the placement of a CVP catheter; namely, the arm (basilic and cephalic vein), the neck (external and internal jugular veins), and the subclavian vein. The first requires the use of an extra long catheter, since the tip must reach the superior vena cava. It is the simplest method and, perhaps, the safest. The external jugular vein may be cannulated either percutaneously or by means of a cutdown. It is sometimes difficult to insert catheters into the subclavian vein from the external jugular because of the angle at which the two vessels meet, but one excellent method of facilitating passage is to ask the patient to turn his head sharply to the contralateral side. An equally effective technique is percutaneous internal jugular catheterization. The fastest and most commonly used method of cannulating the central venous system, however, is direct percutaneous subclavian vein puncture and most of the ensuing discussion refers specifically to this technique.

---

## NEEDED FOR MEASURING CENTRAL VENOUS PRESSURE:

| | |
|---|---|
| Prep sponge and antiseptic | Intravenous tubing set |
| Sterile gloves | 18-inch extension tubing |
| 10-ml syringe | Manometer |
| Percutaneous needle-catheter | Antibiotic ointment |
|    (e.g. Intracath) | Gauze pad and adhesive tape |
| Intravenous fluid | |

---

## Equipment

The subclavian vein may be cannulated with any of the numerous needle-catheter units available today, but a 14-gauge Intracath is preferable (17-gauge for infants). In addition, prep material, antibiotic ointment, adhesive tape, a 10-ml syringe, 18-inch intravenous extension tube, three-way stopcock, and manometer are needed.

## Technique

The infraclavicular approach is used most commonly. Elevate the patient's feet in order to distend the subclavian vein temporarily. Put a pad under the patient's shoulder to lift the clavicle up to widen the space between it and the first rib. Prepare the skin carefully beneath the clavicle with Betadine. Drapes, mask, and sterile gloves should be used. Disassemble a 14-gauge Intracath, carefully set the catheter on the sterile towel, and attach a 10-ml syringe to the needle. Anesthetize the skin with a local anesthetic. Place a small puncture wound in the skin of the chest 2 cm inferior to a point slightly medial to the midpoint of the clavicle using a No. 11 scalpel blade. With the bevel of the needle pointing upward, place the needle through this incision. While maintaining suction on the plunger, keep the syringe parallel to the surface of the chest wall and advance the needle toward the triangular zone which lies between the sternal and clavicular heads of the sternocleidomastoid muscle (Fig. 5.1). The return of dark blood indicates successful puncture of the vein. If the needle strikes the clavicle or fails to enter the vein, withdraw partially and aim slightly deeper. Once in the vein, blood will aspirate freely. Rotate the bevel of the needle 90° toward the feet and ask the patient to inspire deeply and hold his breath (this approximates a Valsalva maneuver). Now remove the syringe and quickly insert the catheter, advancing it about 10 cm. In this way, the threat of air embolism will be diminished. Replace the syringe and make certain that blood returns before connecting the intravenous line. Apply antibiotic ointment to the puncture site and secure the catheter by suturing it to the skin as well as with gauze and tape.

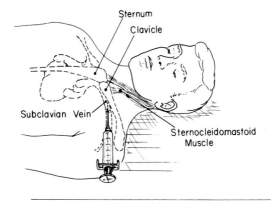

**Figure 5.1.** Infraclavicular approach to subclavian vein. Pierce the skin 2 cm inferior and slightly medial to the midpoint of the clavicle, and then advance the needle toward the triangular zone between the sternal and clavicular heads of the sternocleidomastoid muscle.

The subclavian vein may also be approached from above the clavicle. The needle should pierce the skin at the apex of the angle formed by the superior surface of the clavicle and the lateral border of the sternocleidomastoid muscle. With the needle and syringe held at a 45° angle with the horizontal plane, direct the tip under the clavicle to an average depth of 1½–2 cm. This approach provides less risk of pneumothorax since the needle is directed toward midline and therefore away from the pleural dome.

Success with both the infraclavicular and supraclavicular approaches depends on careful attention to anatomical landmarks. Always use a syringe, because in the event of extremely low venous pressure, blood will not rise spontaneously in the needle and air may be drawn inward. Use only the gentlest aspiration pressure or else the venous walls may collapse. There is ordinarily little or no patient discomfort associated with an indwelling subclavian catheter. Patients must be warned of its importance, however, and asked to avoid any sudden movements which might dislodge the catheter. As a final safety measure, listen to both lung fields afterward to be certain that a pneumothorax has not been produced. Also be alert to the possibility of late development of a pneumothorax. Obtain a chest x-ray soon after the procedure to determine proper placement. Two or three ml of contrast material should be placed down the catheter at the time of the x-ray to determine flow characteristics as well as to better elucidate the placement. The tip of the catheter should be in the midportion of the superior vena cava. If it is too far in, it should be pulled back.

Percutaneous catheterization of the internal jugular vein requires similar positioning and sterile techniques. The face is turned slightly toward the puncture side to relax the sternocleidomastoid muscle. The pulsating common carotid artery is palpated at the medial border of the sternocleidomastoid muscle and the lower border of the thyroid cartilage. One index finger is placed on this artery and the needle is inserted by the other hand lateral to the artery (Fig. 5.2). After the needle is advanced its entire length, the index finger is removed from the artery and the needle is drawn back gradually with negative pressure in the syringe until free flow of blood is obtained indicating that the tip of the needle lies within the lumen of the vein. The syringe is then lowered cephalad to a horizontal position. The syringe is detached from the needle and the catheter is inserted. The internal jugular vein can be entered from posterior to the sternocleidomastoid muscle by turning the head to the side opposite the puncture site (Fig. 5.2).

### Venous Pressure Measurements

In order to use the central venous catheter for fluid infusions and venous pressure measurements, place a three-way valve and an 18-inch extension tube (e.g. Abbott Venotube) in the line. A plastic manometer can be attached to the three-way valve each time a measurement is made, or it may be left in place permanently.

Opinions vary regarding the proper zero mark, and individual anatomical configurations may differ widely as well. Some use the anterior axillary line, others the midaxillary line, and a few carefully measure 3–4 cm below the sternal angle. It is not nearly as important that there be a universal definition of

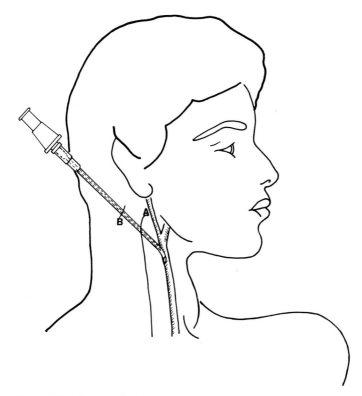

**Figure 5.2.** Internal jugular venipuncture from the anterior (A) and posterior (B) border of sternocleidomastoid muscle. The needle is inserted to its entire length and then it is drawn back slowly until a free flow of blood is obtained in the syringe. The needle is then lowered cephalad for alignment with the vein and insertion of the catheter.

the zero point as it is that everyone caring for a given patient use a single reference point so that all readings will be comparable. Therefore, after inserting the catheter, select your favorite point (e.g. anterior axillary line), place a small strip of adhesive tape on the patient's skin, and ask the nursing staff to use that mark for all future readings. The patient should always be in the same relative position in the bed (e.g. supine and flat).

Assuming that the catheter is fastened well to the chest wall, it is better to allow the manometer to lie freely next to the patient's pillow than to fix it to a metal stand next to the bed where it will have to be adjusted each time the patient's position is changed (Fig. 5.3). Sudden movements by the patient also may dislodge the catheter if the manometer is fixed rigidly.

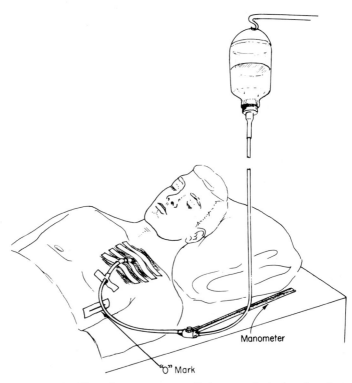

**Figure 5.3.** Allow the manometer to lie loose on the bed, rather than fix it to a pole, so that sudden patient movement will not dislodge the catheter.

Pressure recordings involve the following steps. Place the patient in a supine position and set the base of the manometer next to the premarked zero point on the chest wall. Turn the three-way valve so that the manometer fills with fluid from the bottle. Then turn the valve to a position which allows the subclavian vein to communicate directly with the manometer. The fluid meniscus should fall freely to the level which indicates current pressure and then fluctuate slightly with each inspiration. If it does not, the catheter may be clogged and should be irrigated with sterile saline. After the reading is taken, turn the valve to the third position, which allows for resumption of the infusion. Return the manometer to its position beside the pillow, return the patient to his previous position, and record the pressure on the chart.

A venous pressure transducer can be used in place of the manometer. The transducer should be zeroed at a level similar to the manometer for consistent and meaningful data.

### Interpretation

Normal central venous pressure is considered to lie somewhere within the range of 6–12 cm of $H_2O$, but absolute values are not nearly as important as relative changes in pressure. Many individuals have a perfectly normal pressure of 4 cm. Patients with chronic pulmonary disease and cor pulmonale, on the other hand, may run a chronically elevated venous pressure of 16 cm of $H_2O$ without evidence of cardiac failure. A rapid change from 6 cm to 12 cm (totally within the normal range, incidentally) in a patient receiving intravenous saline may be indicative of early cardiac decompensation.

An absent or unrecordable venous pressure usually indicates contraction of the effective blood volume. A falling central venous pressure may indicate either loss of blood volume (e.g. hemorrhage) or else increased cardiac efficiency (e.g. response to digitalis therapy). A rising central venous pressure indicates filling (perhaps overfilling) of the vascular space or an overloaded heart pumping capacity. This is not universally true, however, since patients in shock can develop pulmonary edema with no elevation of the CVP whatsoever.

The CVP may also be altered by numerous factors which bear no relation to intrinsic heart function. As mentioned before, patients with chronic pulmonary disease have elevations of venous pressure, and therefore CVP monitoring may not be nearly as indicative of the status of the vascular space as in normal persons. Any condition which significantly changes the position of the mediastinum or raises the intrathoracic pressure may also elevate the CVP, e.g. pleural effusion, hemothorax, pneumothorax, chest wall trauma or positive end expiratory pressure (PEEP). Use of the positive pressure breathing apparatus elevates CVP somewhat and should be discontinued briefly before measurement. Any obstruction to cardiac filling, such as cardiac tamponade or superior vena caval obstruction, will necessarily elevate the venous pressure. Any condition that inhibits venous return to the heart, such as ascites or acute gastric dilation, has been shown to decrease CVP and lead to the mistaken impression of hypovolemia.

Despite these shortcomings, CVP monitoring continues to be an extremely useful index. Its true value lies in its sensitivity, since in the presence of hemorrhage the CVP falls before there are detectable alterations of pulse or arterial pressure and, in the presence of incipient cardiac failure, elevation precedes most other signs of decompensation.

## PULMONARY ARTERY CATHETERIZATION

A more accurate assessment of the patient's intravascular volume can be obtained with a Swan-Ganz pulmonary artery catheter. This device permits measurement of the patient's pulmonary artery pressure (PAP), pulmonary capillary wedge pressure (PCWP—an approximation of left atrial pressure) and cardiac output (by thermal dilution technique) (Fig. 5.4). The wedge pressure is a more accurate indicator of intravascular volume than the CVP and can be expected to run near normal levels (10–15 cm water) once resuscitation is adequate.

A thermistor is located in the catheter just proximal to the balloon. Cool saline is injected into the right atrium through

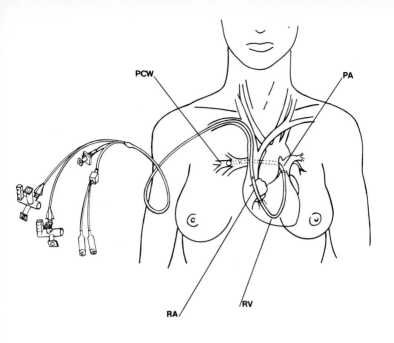

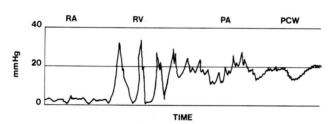

**Figure 5.4.** Swan-Ganz catheter placement. Pressure tracings are depicted as the pulmonary artery catheter is advanced into the right atrium (RA), the right ventrical (RV), the pulmonary artery (PA), and the wedged position (PCW). As the catheter is passed, the appearance of the pressure tracing indicates the position of the catheter. The RAP and the PCWP showed two elevations per cardiac cycle and the RVP and PAP only one. The PAP is differentiated from the RVP by the elevated diastolic baseline. Advance a little further into the wedge position and the tracings should show a much lower pressure which should have an atrial form. It may be necessary to deflate the balloon, advance 2–3 cm and reinflate the balloon.

a separate lumen opening 30 cm proximal to the balloon. Mixing takes place in the right ventricle and the temperature curve traced by the thermistor is used to calculate the cardiac output. Computers are available that will measure the temperature of the injected saline, monitor the thermistor, perform the calculations automatically, and display the cardiac output on a digital readout.

Left ventricular performance can be estimated from the PCWP and cardiac output. This technique is useful for monitoring acutely ill patients with known pre-existent cardiac disease, respiratory failure, and massive fluid and electrolyte replacement requirements.

The catheter may be placed by cutdown or by the Seldinger percutaneous technique at any of the sites recommended for CVP. Strict aseptic conditions must be observed for insertion and management. Using the Seldinger technique, a peripheral or central vein is cannulated, a wound spring-type wire is passed through the cannula, and the cannula is removed. A dilator and an introducing sleeve are passed over the guide wire. The dilator and the wire are removed and the Swan-Ganz catheter can be passed through the sleeve into the vein. The distal lumen of the catheter is attached to a venous pressure transducer and monitor and pressures are measured continually throughout the catherization procedure (Fig. 5.4). The tip balloon is inflated (0.5–1.5 ml air) when the catheter is in the right atrium and the catheter is flow-directed through the right heart into the pulmonary artery (Fig. 5.4). As a check on position, connect the pressure gauge to the proximal lumen. This should show a right atrial pressure curve. If it shows a right ventricular pressure, the catheter is in too far and should be pulled back. If cardiac index and flow are low, it may be difficult to pass the catheter and several attempts may be necessary. Catheter position is always confirmed by x-ray (Fig. 5.5).

## Complications

Pneumothorax stands as the most frequent and most serious complication of subclavian puncture. Its reported incidence

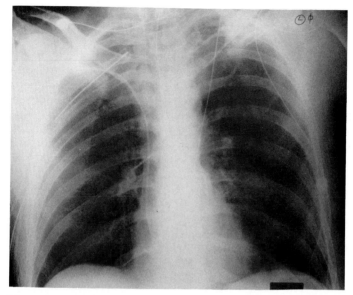

**Figure 5.5.** Posteroanterior (PA) chest roentgenogram of Swan-Ganz catheter placement. Distal tip of catheter is in the pulmonary artery.

lies somewhere between 0.2 and 2%. It more commonly follows infra-clavicular puncture, particularly when the needle is inserted too deeply and too far laterally. Dyspnea, chest pain, or unequal breath sounds following subclavian puncture calls for prompt chest x-ray and a chest tube if necessary.

Although failure to enter the subclavian vein is usually a result of inexperience, a certain number of patients defy successful puncture because of obesity or unusual anatomy. In any event, it is more prudent to resort to a cutdown (e.g. cephalic or external jugular vein) rather than attempt to puncture both sides and risk producing a bilateral pneumothorax.

Thrombophlebitis is rare following subclavian tap, although it occurs occasionally after external jugular, basilic, or cephalic vein cannulation. This low incidence is probably related to the increased flow rates in the subclavian vein, as well as the fact that the catheter floats freely within the wide lumen and does not become fixed to the wall as it does in smaller veins.

Swan-Ganz catheterization has been complicated by mural thrombosis in the right ventricle with subsequent staphylococcal infection and bacterial endocarditis. Moreover, thrombosis at the subclavian catheterization site with subsequent sustained staphylococcal bacteremia has occurred.

Although small amounts of air may enter the subclavian vein during cannulation, this is not usually harmful (except in patients with septal defects). Air entry can be minimized by 1) using the Trendelenburg position, 2) asking the patient to hold his breath during catheter insertion, and 3) moving quickly. In the event of massive air embolism, the patient should be turned promptly on his *left side* to avoid pulmonary embolism.

Cardiac tamponade has been reported following advancement of the subclavian catheter into the right ventricle where, after several days, its tip eroded into the pericardial sac. CVP catheters need never be passed beyond the superior vena cava for accurate pressure measurement.

Malposition of the catheter (i.e. internal carotid artery) can occur and must be corrected promptly—thus, the reason for a chest x-ray with contrast material infusion.

The Swan-Ganz catheter has some additional unique complications. Occasionally, the catheter causes persistent premature ventricular contractions. These usually respond to Lidocaine. Rupture of the balloon usually produces no ill effects except that no PCWP measurement is possible. Intracardiac twisting and/or knotting of the catheter occurs when excess catheter is advanced too rapidly. Pulmonary artery erosion, interpulmonary wedging, and pulmonary embolus may also occur.

Finally, central venous catheters, and in particular the pulmonary artery catheters, should be removed as soon as possible when they are no longer needed for monitoring the acutely ill patient. It is not desirable to leave a pulmonary artery catheter in place longer than 72 hours.

## Selected References for Further Reading

1. Brisman, R., Parks, L. C., and Benson, D. W. Pitfalls in the clinical use of central venous pressure. *Arch. Surg. (Chicago) 95:* 902–907, 1967.
2. Central venous pressure (editorial). *J.A.M.A. 202:* 1099, 1967.
3. DeFalque, R. J. Subclavian venipuncture: A review. *Anesth. Anal. (Cleveland) 47:* 677–682, 1968.
4. Kline, I. K. and Hofman, W. I. Cardiac tamponade from CVP catheter perforation. *J.A.M.A. 206:* 1794–1795, 1968.
5. Longerbeam, J. K., Vannia, R., Wagner, W., and Joergenson, E. Central venous pressure monitoring. *Amer. J. Surg. 110:* 220–230, 1965.
6. Parsa, M. H., Farrer, J. M., and Habif, D. V. Safe central venous nutrition. Springfield, Ill. Charles C Thomas, 1974.
7. Swan, H. J. C., Ganz, W., Forrester, J., Marcus, H., Diamond, G., and Chonette, D. Catheterization of the heart in man with use of a flow-directed balloon-tipped catheter. *New Eng. J. Med. 283:* 447, 1970.
8. Swan, H. J. C. Balloon flotation catheters: their use in hemodynamic monitoring in clinical practice. *J.A.M.A. 233:* 865, 1975.
9. Wilson, J. N., Grow, J. B., DeMong, C. V., Prevedel, A. E., and Owens, J. C. Central venous pressure in optimal blood volume maintenance. *Arch. Surg. (Chicago) 85:* 563–578, 1962.

## SIX

# Other Injection Techniques

Routes of parenteral drug administration are named according to the tissue layer into which the medication is injected. This chapter deals with three such routes, "intradermal," "subcutaneous," and "intramuscular" (Fig. 6.1). Intravenous injections are considered independently under venipuncture.

## INTRADERMAL

This method is used almost exclusively for determining patient sensitivity to medications. Skin testing may be used to determine allergies, identify tuberculosis exposure, and predict adverse reactions to drugs or local anesthetics.

The volar aspect of the forearm is used most frequently. When it becomes necessary to carry out a large number of injections, the back offers an ideal surface. Careful attention to technique must be observed or the test results will be meaningless. The volume to be injected should not exceed 0.2 ml. A 25-gauge short needle is appropriate. Small tuberculin or insulin syringes facilitate precise measurement of volume injected. Hold the arm firmly and draw the skin taut between thumb and forefinger. Hold the needle (bevel up) and syringe nearly parallel to the skin surface and insert the tip just beneath the epithelium. If the needle is well placed, a pale white raised zone should develop as the test substance is injected. Bleeding should always be absent! If blood appears, make note of it since the presence of ecchymosis may render the reading (usu-

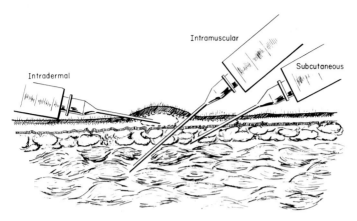

**Figure 6.1.** Three common methods of injection.

ally 48 hours later) uninterpretable. Always record in the patient's chart which tests were done, when, and the exact location of each.

## SUBCUTANEOUS

A subcutaneous (or "hypodermic") injection means literally "under the skin." The drug is deposited within the fat but above the muscle. When accurately placed, nerve injury is rarely a danger and there is a wide choice of acceptable injection sites. The outer surface of the upper arm or anterior surface of the thigh are selected most commonly. Diabetics who must learn to rotate their injection sites will, in addition, use the abdomen. There are several factors which influence the selection of the subcutaneous route for drug administration. The subcutaneous injection site affords rapid absorption but the onset of drug action depends upon the density of blood vessels in the area of injection.

First, select the appropriate syringe and needle. Draw up the medication making certain to release any air caught within the syringe. Up to 5 ml may be administered in a single injection. Prepare the skin over the injection site with an antiseptic.

While holding the skin flat and moderately tense, insert the needle firmly and rapidly at a 45° angle until a sudden release signifies penetration of the dermis. Draw back on the syringe to make certain a blood vessel hasn't been pierced; then inject slowly. Following withdrawal of the needle, rub the skin briskly with a sponge to stimulate circulation, promote distribution of the drug, and alleviate discomfort.

Alternately, pinch up the subcutaneous tissue into a roll and inject at a slight angle to the base of the raised tissue. This assures placement of the drug deep in the fat but above the muscular layer. Release the skin following insertion of the needle to prevent painful injection under pressure.

# INTRAMUSCULAR

Intramuscular injection is the route of choice for drugs which cannot be easily absorbed from the subcutaneous layer. Examples include penicillin and steroids. In addition, larger drug volumes can be given by this route; as much as 10 cc in carefully chosen sites.

Some controversy prevails regarding the best site for intramuscular injection. The gluteal region is used most commonly, but if care is not taken, nerve injury may result. Four alternative sites are compared here:

## Deltoid Muscle

This should not be equated with "upper arm" since the safe zone includes only the main body of the deltoid muscle lying lateral and a few centimeters beneath the acromion. There is little threat of radial nerve injury unless the needle strays into the middle or lower third of the arm. This site will accept only small volumes, e.g. less than 2 cc. The deltoid is the injection site of choice in patients with chronic congestive heart failure since there may be no effective drug absorption from edematous buttock muscles.

### Gluteal Region

This should not be considered synonymous with "buttock"! The greatest danger here is the inadvertent injury to the sciatic nerve. Furthermore, the superior gluteal artery courses through the same region. Another disadvantage of this site is that an abundance of subcutaneous fat can prevent the needle from reaching the muscle! Deposition of large drug volumes into fat is a distinct error since absorption is slower, pain is more severe, and the chance of fat necrosis or sterile abscess formation is very real.

Nonetheless, the gluteal region remains the most commonly used injection site. However, its satisfactory use depends on cautious technique. Only the upper outer buttock quadrant, farthest from the nerve and artery should be used (Fig. 6.2).

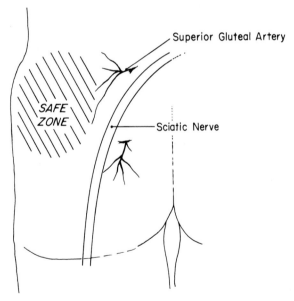

**Figure 6.2.** Gluteal injections must be restricted to the upper outer quadrant in order to avoid injury to the sciatic nerve.

Draw back on the syringe before injecting the drug to make certain that a blood vessel has not been entered. *Never* persist with an injection that produces radicular leg pain.

### Lateral Thigh (Vastus Lateralis Muscle)

This is perhaps the safest injection site because there are few, if any, arteries or nerves nearby. In addition, this muscle will accept large drug volumes, i.e. 10 cc. Perhaps the only disadvantage of this site is the firm fascia lata overlying the muscle which makes needle insertion somewhat more painful.

### Pectoral Muscle

A muscle rarely used but perfectly safe is the pectoralis major. In patients whose other sites have been overused, the entire anterior axillary fold can be grasped between fingers and thumb and considerable drug injected into the available muscle mass.

## COMPLICATIONS

Nerve and arterial injury have already been listed as potential complications of intramuscular injection. In addition, abscesses, both sterile and septic, may arise from careless technique or overuse of a specific injection site.

The mechanism of nerve injury is poorly understood. In the past, the properties of the drug have commonly been blamed for the neuritis that follows. It is recognized now that even sterile saline might produce nerve sheath inflammation, muscle wasting, weakness, or paralysis. In fact, the nerve does not even have to be touched. A hematoma which encircles the nerve can produce irreversible injury. Most agree, however, that neural injury can be minimized by prudent selection and rotation of injection sites.

## Selected References for Further Reading

1. Bailey, H. Hollow-needle technique in injection therapy. In *Pye's Surgical Handicraft,* Vol. 1. Williams & Wilkins, Baltimore, 1962, pp. 56–68.
2. Broadbent, T. R., Odom, G. L., and Woodhall, B. Peripheral nerve injuries from administration of penicillin. *J.A.M.A. 140:* 1008–1010, 1949.
3. Gilles, F. H. and French, J. H. Post-injection sciatic nerve palsies in infants and children. *J. Pediat. 58:* 195–204, 1961.
4. Hansen, D. J. Intramuscular injection injuries and complications. *GP 27:* 109–115, 1963.
5. Turner, G. G. The site for intramuscular injections. *Lancet 2:* 819, 1920.

# SEVEN

# Pulmonary Care

The principles of first aid dictate that, in the event of an accident, the highest priority must be given to respiratory function. Likewise, the already hospitalized patient must always be given the very best respiratory care. Two patient groups in particular require specific procedures designed for this purpose: those with cardiopulmonary disease and those in the early postoperative period whose painful incisions prevent them from inspiring and coughing adequately. This chapter discusses some of these clinical techniques.

## COUGHING

No mechanical device can substitute for the persistent urging of a patient to take deep breaths and cough. Effective coughing demands proper positioning. In theory, the bronchial passages should drain best with the head down and the feet elevated— and they do, but this is often impractical and causes breathing difficulty because the diaphragm must move against the weight of the abdominal contents. Patients usually cough best in an upright position. Frequent turning from side to side also prevents retention of secretions.

Painful incisions are the greatest inhibitors of coughing. Analgesia in moderate doses is, therefore, an essential part of good pulmonary care. It is just as wrong to withhold all narcotics as it is to depress the patient with unnecessarily large doses.

Many patients will not cough on their own and must be coaxed persistently and frequently. Although bracing the incision with the hands is helpful, a far more effective measure is to hold each lateral rib cage with moderate pressure as coughing takes place. In the case of an abdominal incision, the cough impulse will then be transmitted to the assisting hands rather than to the incision, thus diminishing pain. A folded pillow held firmly against the abdomen by the patient also decreases discomfort. Remember also to provide tissues for the patient when urging him to cough, for it is surprisingly easier to develop a strong cough if a target for potential secretions is in view!

## INHALATION THERAPY

A number of respiratory aids are available which provide one or more of the following benefits: 1) augmented oxygen concentrations, 2) humidity, and 3) positive pressure breathing support. Far too often importance is placed upon providing extra oxygen while at the same time directing little attention to humidification.

Oxygen may be delivered in numerous ways, each with inherent disadvantages as well as differing degrees of efficiency. A catheter may be advanced into the oral pharynx so that the tip lies just visible beside the uvula (Fig. 7.1). With flows of 6–8 liters/minute, oxygen concentrations of 35–40% may be delivered. If a catheter is placed merely in the nose, then very little benefit will be achieved at the capillary-alveolar level as the patient breathes through the mouth. If the catheter is passed too far, it may enter the esophagus and produce gastric distention. A suitable guide is to insert a length of catheter no greater than the distance from the tip of the nose to the tragus of the ear. Transnasal catheters are simple and acceptable to most patients, but oxygen given in this manner may have a severe drying effect on the respiratory mucosa. Therefore, a source of humidity should always be included in the oxygen line.

An oxygen tent usually provides no greater oxygen concen-

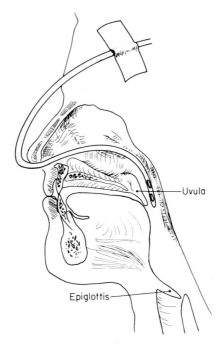

**Figure 7.1.** The tip of an intranasal oxygen catheter should lie behind the uvula.

tration to the patient than a transnasal catheter. Its efficiency is quite dependent upon the care which is taken in sealing the plastic enclosure with the bed linen. A major disadvantage of tents is their tendency to separate the patient from medical and nursing personnel. Patients confined within them also experience depression and a feeling of abandonment.

Loosely fitting facial masks with mixing holes deliver at least as much oxygen (35–50%) as the nasal catheter. Higher concentrations of oxygen (>50%) and constant positive airway pressure (CPAP) require a closed system, i.e. a tight fitting silastic face mask. Patients who need respiratory assistance in addition to $O_2$ require either endotracheal intubation or a cuffed tracheostomy tube.

Regarding the need for humidity, it is pertinent to recall that an intact respiratory tract loses 8–10 gm of $H_2O$/cubic m of air expired. Most of this loss is returned during inspiration. However, when there is an excess loss of $H_2O$ content, severe imbalances soon occur. Nothing will thicken secretions more effectively than dehydration, either local or systemic! Marked deficits of inspired water produce squamous metaplasia of the respiratory epithelium, particularly in patients with tracheostomies or endotracheal tubes who have lost their entire water-conserving apparatus. Moisture is essential, therefore, preferably administered by a nebulizer. Warm humidity is preferable to cold humidity, since warm air holds more moisture than cold air.

Intermittent use of positive pressure support (IPPB) is beneficial for the administration of bronchodilator agents. Chronic pulmonary disease victims, of course, must rely heavily on periodic use of these machines. Both the Bird and Bennett respirators (as well as other varieties) allow for the administration of humidity, mucolytic agents, and oxygen.

A variety of incentive spirometers (Fig. 7.2A) can be used to improve pulmonary function. Such support should not be reserved for the moribund individual. Intermittent use (10–20 minute periods) every 2 hours is beneficial for preoperative as well as postoperative patients. Blow bottles in which the patient must displace colored water from one bottle to another will serve as an inexpensive substitute for the incentive spirometer based on the observation that a patient must take in a deep breath before he can breathe out (Fig. 7.2B).

## TRACHEAL SUCTION

Whenever the physician is faced with an uncooperative patient, or when the measures discussed thus far have failed to prevent fever and pulmonary atelectasis, then more aggressive methods must be applied. Tracheal suction becomes necessary any time that the patient cannot keep his lungs clear by spontaneous or stimulated coughing.

In addition to an adequate suction apparatus, a Y connector

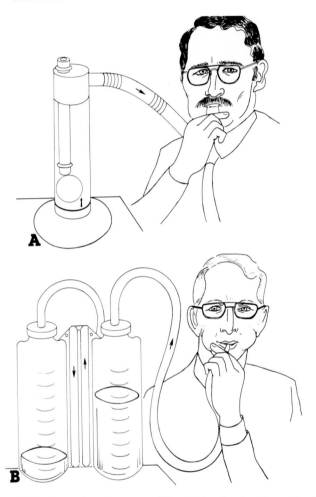

**Figure 7.2.** Incentive spirometers (**A**) and blow bottles (**B**) are simple to explain and use.

should be interposed between the main tubing and the tracheal catheter. Although strict sterile technique is difficult to maintain, its application is nevertheless mandatory in order to prevent tracheal or bronchial contamination. Always wear clean plastic gloves in order to avoid catheter contamination. Replace the catheter every time that it is used.

With the patient sitting upright, extend the head and grasp the tip of the tongue with a gauze pad (Fig. 7.3). This prevents swallowing, elevates the epiglottis, and allows the catheter to enter the trachea more easily. As the patient inhales, introduce a catheter lubricated with Lidocaine jelly transnasally. Entrance into the trachea will usually be heralded by a paroxysm of coughing. Then ask the patient to quiet down, keep breath-

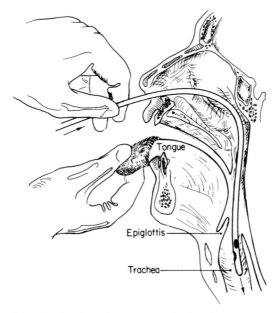

**Figure 7.3.** Tracheal suction: extend the head, grasp the tongue, and ask the patient to inspire as the catheter is advanced.

ing, and refrain from speaking. Once the catheter has entered the trachea, leave it there for the duration of the procedure.

Now connect the catheter to the suction source and occlude the Y connector with your thumb, thus diverting all suction to the tip. Periods of aspiration must be brief (5–10 seconds) and intermittent (every 25–30 seconds) or asphyxia will occur. A few milliliters (2–3) of saline may be introduced into the mainstem bronchi, if desired, in order to induce better coughing.

A special word of precaution is warranted in view of the many reports of cardiac arrest following overzealous tracheal suction. The cause appears to be associated with vagal stimulation of acutely hypoxic and hypercarbic patients. Therefore, brief and intermittent periods of suction are of paramount importance. One effective method for limiting the suction period is to occlude the Y connector only as long as you can hold your own breath comfortably.

## PERCUTANEOUS POLYETHYLENE TUBE TRACHEOSTOMY

A technique which has earned popular support is the introduction of a small catheter percutaneously through the cricothyroid membrane to provide a better route for instillation of saline into the trachea. A 17-gauge Bard Intracath is suitable and can be inserted under local anesthesia. Advance the catheter about 7 cm into the trachea and then tape it in place. Periodic instillation of saline (2 ml) serves as a reliable cough stimulus for 1–2 days.

Indications for this technique include major surgery with anticipated respiratory difficulty, unwillingness of the patient to cough, or inability to obtain a sample of sputum for culture. This procedure is contraindicated in the absence of cough reflex or in asthma patients who might experience bronchospasm. The technique may be used in place of tracheal suction, but it should not be considered a substitute for tracheostomy.

Complications are rare if the cricothyroid membrane is used.

When piercing a tracheal ring one runs the risk of causing hemorrhage by damaging the thyroid isthmus. Subcutaneous emphysema has also developed after lower sites of introduction are used. At either site, one must be extremely cautious to secure the tube well so that patients cannot inhale the catheter into the trachea.

# OTHER MEASURES

The patient who cannot be helped with tracheal suction usually requires bronchoscopy or tracheostomy.

### Selected References for Further Reading

1. Bartlett, R. H., Gazzaniga, A. B., and Geraghty, T. R. Respiratory maneuvers to prevent post-operative pulmonary complications: a critical review. *J.A.M.A. 224:* 1017–1021, 1973.
2. Fineburg, C., Cohn, H. E., and Gibbon, J. H. Cardiac arrest during nasotracheal aspiration. *J.A.M.A. 174:* 410–412, 1960.
3. Haight, C. Intratracheal suction in the management of post-operative pulmonary complications. *Ann. Surg. 107:* 218–288, 1938.
4. Moore, F. D. Oxygen toxicity as a factor, discussion of a paper by Pratt, P. C., *J. Trauma 8:* 865, 1968.
5. Myers, R. N., Shearburn, E. W., and Haupt, G. J. Prevention and management of pulmonary complications by percutaneous polyethylene tube tracheostomy. *Amer. J. Surg. 109:* 590–593, 1965.
6. Sara, C. and Currie, T. Humidification by nebulization. *Med. J. Aust. 1:* 174–179, 1965.
7. Segal, M. S. Treatment of acute respiratory failure. *New Eng. J. Med. 274:* 841–844, 1966.
8. Van de Water, J. M., Watring, W. G., Linton, L. A., Murphy, M. and Byron, R. L. Prevention of post-operative pulmonary complications. *Surg. Gynec. Obstet. 135:* 229–235, 1972.
9. Wolstad, P. M. and Conklin, W. S. Rupture of the normal stomach after therapeutic oxygen administration. *New Eng. J. Med. 264:* 1201–1202, 1961.

# EIGHT

# Thoracentesis

The term thoracentesis is derived from two Greek words, *"thorakos,"* meaning that portion of the body covered by the breastbone, and *"kenteo,"* meaning to pierce. It simply refers to the introduction of a needle into the pleural space. Thoracentesis may be performed for a number of reasons, among them drainage of fluid accumulations, re-expansion of a lung compressed by an air-filled pleural space, or for removal of a specimen needed for diagnostic examination. In addition, this chapter includes a brief discussion of pericardiocentesis.

## EQUIPMENT

Chest tap trays usually contain gauze pads and antiseptic for preping, sterile drapes, and a 10-ml syringe with a 22-gauge (long) and a 25-gauge (short) needle for anesthesia. The chest is tapped with an 18-gauge short bevel needle and 50-ml syringe. In addition, a three-way stopcock, rubber tubing, and a hemostat are necessary to aid in controlling steady fluid aspiration. Finally, a large sterile metal basin as well as two to three glass tubes are needed for the aspirate. The procedure may be simplified and much of the aforementioned equipment made unnecessary if a sterile vacuum bottle unit is available. However, one sacrifices a certain degree of control over suction force so that use of these units is best limited to patients with large chronic effusions.

## NEEDED FOR A CHEST TAP:

| | |
|---|---|
| Prep sponges and antiseptic | Three-way stopcock |
| Sterile towels | Rubber tubing |
| 22- and 25-gauge needles | Hemostatic clamp |
| 10-ml syringe | Sterile metal basin |
| Local anesthetic (1% Lidocaine) | Three specimen tubes |
| 18-gauge short bevel needle | Vacuum bottle (optional) |
| 50-ml syringe | |

## TECHNIQUE

Before beginning, it is wise to review several essential anatomical facts (Fig. 8.1). Anterior to the midaxillary line, there are two neurovascular bundles in each intercostal space. Therefore, needles or trocars should be placed between the ribs or in midinterspace. Posterior to the midaxillary line, there is but one bundle, and it lies just beneath the lower costal margin. Therefore, needles should be inserted at the bottom of the interspace, i.e. just above the margin of the inferior rib.

If air is to be removed, the second intercostal space anteriorly is the preferred site. However, if the goal is fluid drainage, a more posterior and dependent location is appropriate. A recent chest x-ray is the best guide to where the fluid is located. Usually, however, the sixth interspace is used. The lower tip of the scapula can serve as a reference point since it usually overlies the seventh rib or seventh interspace. If the sixth intercostal space is selected, ask the patient to raise his arms (i.e. rest them on an attendant's shoulders or bedstand), so that this site will be accessible. A good general rule is to avoid inserting anything below the fourth rib anteriorly, sixth rib laterally, or eighth rib posteriorly lest damage be inflicted on visceral organs beneath the diaphragm. This is particularly

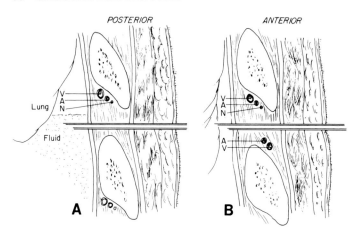

**Figure 8.1.** A, posterior to the midaxillary line, the needles should pass over the superior surface of the inferior rib. B, anterior to the midaxillary line, the needle should pass through the middle of the interspace.

true when the patient is lying down or when there is poor inspiration.

The patient should be sitting with both legs over the edge of the bed, arms resting on a bed table (Fig. 8.2). If there is any danger that the patient will move suddenly or fall, ask an assistant to stand by the bed and provide support. Standing behind the patient, select the desired interspace and make a small indentation in the skin with the edge of your fingernail. This prevents the necessity of recounting ribs later on. Prepare the skin widely around the site including an extra interspace above and below. Next, arrange drapes below the selected interspace and on the bed in order to provide a working space. Omit drapes above the injection site for they serve no real function and might fall as the patient moves.

Fill the syringe with local anesthetic (1% Lidocaine) and raise an intradermal wheal at the previously marked site. Switch to a 22-gauge (long) needle and infiltrate the intercostal

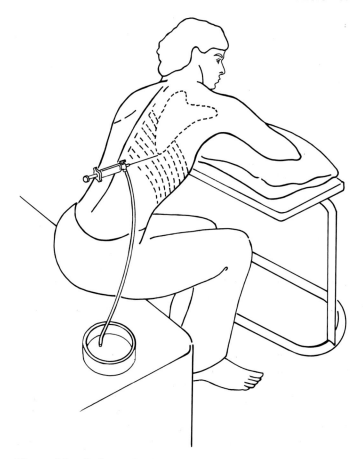

**Figure 8.2.** Patients should be sitting upright but resting on a bedstand during thoracentesis.

muscles. It is sometimes possible to advance farther and find the pleural space before switching to the larger thoracentesis needle if the pleura is not thickened excessively. Withdraw and wait at least 5 minutes (look at your watch!) for the anesthetic to take effect. Meanwhile, attach the syringe, three-way stop-cock, and 18-gauge needle in one assembly and advance slowly along the infiltrated tract. Remember to stay low, passing just above the inferior rib margin. Don't "bounce" the needle over the bone surface since the rib periosteum is quite tender and this is very painful. By maintaining back pressure on the syringe, entrance into the pleural space will be heralded by the sudden return of fluid. A distinct release can be felt as the needle pierces the pleura. After the pleura is entered, place a hemostat on the needle flush with the skin surface to prevent further movement. Now connect the rubber tubing to the three-way valve. Fluid can be removed in 50-ml aliquots with the syringe and repeatedly emptied through the side arm of the stopcock into a sterile basin. Fluid samples should be collected for *routine* bacterial, fungus, and acid-fast bacillus culture, as well as smear, cell count, and cell block (for tumor cells). If fluid cannot be found at one interspace, try another.

If red frothy material appears in the syringe or the patient begins to cough violently, this indicates lung puncture and the needle should be withdrawn at once. In such an event, observe the patient closely for respiratory distress and obtain a chest x-ray in order to determine whether a pneumothorax has developed.

Large effusions are a special problem. Opinions vary regarding the maximum amount of fluid which can be safely removed at one time, but 1000 ml seems to be a reasonable limit. Multiple daily taps are preferable to draining an effusion larger than this in one stage since shock due to rapid fluid shifts may accompany excessive aspirations. In addition, patients cannot comfortably tolerate removal of much more than one liter of fluid at one time.

After a successful chest tap, remove the needle and ask the patient to lie down and rest. Label the specimens and send them off to the laboratory promptly. A descriptive note should then be placed in the patient's chart. If several sites have been tried, the best locations should be marked clearly (e.g. methylene blue or skin marker) for future reference.

# SPECIAL PROBLEMS

## Chronic Effusion

Many advocate the insertion of a catheter (e.g. Intracath or Angiocath) within the pleural space in order to provide continuous drainage and avoid multiple taps. This technique is useful when removing a transudate, but the narrow catheters quickly become occluded by exudates. Catheters are best used after an initial thoracentesis has been carried out and a satisfactory interspace found for drainage. After 2–3 days, however, they represent a potential source of pleural contamination and should be removed or replaced.

## Empyema

If the pus is thick, an 18-gauge needle may be too small in diameter, thus giving a false negative top. Moreover, simple needle aspiration of an infected pleural collection does not ensure adequate drainage. A large bore tube must be inserted or, preferable, a closed chest tube thoracostomy. Later, a partial rib resection may be necessary.

## Effusion Secondary to Subdiaphragmatic Abscess

In the event of coexistent pleural effusion and subdiaphragmatic abscess, there is a very real danger of converting the sterile effusion into an empyema cavity by simultaneously piercing both the pleura and the diaphragm. Therefore, be alert to the possibility of a subdiaphragmatic abscess, in which case thoracentesis should be avoided. If a diagnostic tap is necessary, then enter as high as is practical in order to avoid the already elevated diaphragm. Acute pancreatitis can cause a left pleural effusion also.

## Pleural Biopsy

A biopsy of the pleura can be performed at the time of the initial thoracentesis by using the Cope needle. The biopsy should be done before the pleural effusion is drained since use of this needle is less safe in the absence of an effusion.

The Cope needle has three parts. The outer portion is 11-gauge and has a small screw clamp on it to allow adjustment of the depth to which the needle passes. The two smaller inner portions are an obturator needle for insertion and a hook designed to snare a small piece of tissue for diagnosis upon removal (Fig. 8.3).

Prepare and drape the skin of the chest as for a thoracentesis. Make a small nick in the skin with a No. 11 blade to allow passage of the cannula and obturator needle. Remove the obturator and aspirate fluid to determine whether the needle is in the chest. Set the screw clamp next to the skin and tighten it. Holding the outer cannula, pull the needle out and replace it with the hooked biopsy needle. Pull the outer cannula back far enough so that its tip is outside the pleural cavity and pull the hook back slowly pressing gently in the direction of the hook. Engage the pleura with the hook (Fig. 8.3). After engag-

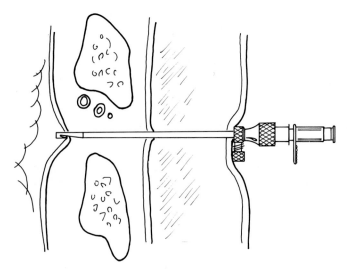

**Figure 8.3.** Pleural biopsy with Cope needle.

ing the pleura with the hook, advance the outer cannula over the cutting edge, snipping off a pleural specimen. Withdraw the whole assembly and remove the piece of pleura. This procedure may be performed several times to obtain sufficient tissue.

## COMPLICATIONS

Hemorrhage from intercostal vessels may occur if heed is not paid to the anatomical position of blood vessels in the interspace. This is particularly important during pleural biopsies. In addition, the splenic capsule or liver may be torn if the procedure is performed in a cavalier fashion at too low a level. A drop in blood pressure after thoracentesis requires a prompt portable chest x-ray and careful abdominal examination.

Pneumothorax should be an infrequent complication of a chest tap. It may follow inadvertent injection of air, but more commonly the needle tip simply lacerates the lung parenchyma after it has been introduced too far. If you suspect that air has entered the pleural cavity, order a chest x-ray. Ordinarily, a pneumothorax following thoracentesis is minimal and requires no specific treatment. However, the threat of tension pneumothorax exists and the nursing staff must be alerted to its possibility. Any sizable pneumothorax producing symptoms or the development of a tension pneumothorax calls for prompt insertion of a chest tube.

Air embolism has been reported following thoracentesis, apparently following injection of air into a peripleural pulmonary vein. This is probably the basis for "pleural shock," once a popular diagnosis. Careful attention to technique, however, should allow one to avoid this tragic complication completely.

## PERICARDIOCENTESIS

Although rarely performed, pericardiocentesis may be a lifesaving procedure in the presence of pericardial tamponade.

This event is often heralded by Beck's triad: i.e. diminished heart sounds, weak or absent pulse, and severely distended neck veins. An elevated CVP supports the diagnosis. There are two commonly used approaches to the pericardial sac, left parasternal and subcostal. The first is least preferred since one risks laceration of the lung as well as the possibility of injuring a major branch of the coronary vessels.

The subcostal approach is far superior, since it is easiest and there is little chance of striking other vital structures. Introduce a cardiac needle between the xyphoid and lower edge of the costal margin (Fig. 8.4). Advance superiorly with the needle

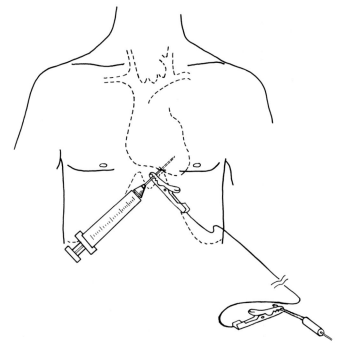

**Figure 8.4.** Pericardiocentesis can be performed most easily by the subcostal-paraxyphoid approach. A wire with double alligator clips may be used to connect the needle to an EKG monitor.

aimed toward the middle of the left axilla. Maintain back pressure on the plunger until a flow of blood enters the syringe. In the presence of tamponade, this will occur as the needle enters the pericardial sac. There should be no air in the syringe. To monitor that the needle hasn't penetrated the myocardium, the limb leads of the EKG should be placed on the legs and the chest lead should be connected to the pericardiocentesis needle. This is manifest by the great increase in voltage or so-called injury current. It is not necessary to drain this space since removal of 100–150 ml of blood or fluid will result in a dramatic return of circulation. Pericardiocentesis may need to be repeated more than once until the source of bleeding is controlled in the operating room. Many people believe that a second pericardiocentesis is a strict indication for thoracotomy. One way to be certain that pericardial blood has been aspirated is to examine it for clots. Heart action ordinarily defibrinates blood in the pericardial space so that it will not clot.

Another procedure calling for this technique is intracardiac drug injection. In this case, the needle must be inserted almost to the needle hub. Blood must be aspirated into the syringe before injecting drugs or else intramural instillation may produce an arrhythmia.

### Selected References for Further Reading

1. Bougas, J. A. Cardiac tamponade. *Surg. Clin. N. Amer. 46:* 563–572, 1966.
2. Carr, D. T. Diagnostic studies of pleural fluid. *Surg. Clin. N. Amer. 53:* 801–804, 1973.
3. Cope, C. and Bernhardt, H. Hook-needle biopsy of pleura, pericardium, peritoneum, and synovium. *Amer. J. Med. 35:* 189–195, 1963.
4. Gibbon, J. H. *Surgery of the Chest.* W. B. Saunders, Philadelphia, 1962, p. 230.
5. Gott, P. H. A simplified method for thoracentesis and pleural fluid drainage. *Amer. Rev. Resp. Dis. 92:* 295–296, 1965.
6. Light, R. W., McGregor, I., Luchsinger, P. C., and Ball, W. C. Pleural effusion: the diagnosis separation of transudates and exudates. *Ann. Intern. Med. 77:* 507–513, 1972.
7. Scerbo, J., Keltz, H., and Stone, D. J. A prospective study of closed pleural biopsies. *J.A.M.A. 218:* 377–380, 1971.

# NINE

# Closed Chest Tube Thoracostomy

Chest tubes, chest drainage bottles, their installation, and their maintenance traditionally has confounded medical students, nurses, and physicians alike. Yet, the importance of thoracostomy cannot be over emphasized, and the technique and principles upon which it is based should be studied carefully. Whenever the integrity of the chest wall or lung surface is interrupted, whether this be spontaneous or traumatic, air escapes into the pleural space, the lung begins to collapse, and the mediastinum shifts toward the unaffected side. This clinical event, called pneumothorax, may be life-threatening, particularly in those instances where the site of air leakage functions as a one-way valve, forcing air into the pleural space but preventing its escape (tension pneumothorax). Both problems call for prompt insertion of a chest tube connected to an underwater seal in order to provide for drainage of the escaped air and re-expansion of the lung.

## HISTORY

The gravity of sucking chest wounds has been recognized by soldiers and military surgeons alike throughout history. A classic description was recorded during the Battle of Mantinea in 362 B.C., during which Epaminondas was pierced in the chest with a spear. Knowing of the certain fatal outcome, he deliberately postponed removal of the spear until he learned of his army's victory. A rush of air was heard soon after the missle was dislodged and death soon overcame him.

Despite numerous similar observations recorded by a variety of military historians, it was not until 1767 that a physiologist, William Hewson, performed animal experiments which proved that pneumothorax was invariably accompanied by air in the pleural cavity. Soon thereafter, Laennec described the clinical features of spontaneous pneumothorax, but made no mention of treatment.

Experience during the Revolutionary War did not result in any new thoughts on the matter. One surgeon's memoirs describes a patient with a sucking wound whose consulting surgeon recommended only bloodletting. Like other afflictions, venesection served as the treatment of choice for chest wounds in that era, since it was readily observed by all surgeons that hemorrhage and air escape were dramatically diminished if enough blood was removed (while the patient lapsed into shock and respiratory depression).

The development of chest tubes and water seal drainage took place in 1875, when Bulan applied these devices to drainage of empyema cavities. Even at the outset of World War I, however, chest wounds were not routinely closed or drained. Dr. Evarts Graham demonstrated that the mediastinum was totally mobile and eventually convinced other surgeons to use the tube thoracostomy initially until thick pus had occurred before employing open drainage. By the end of the war, most surgeons had learned that open or closed pneumothorax could be treated successfully by the institution of thoracostomy and closed underwater seal drainage.

---

## NEEDED FOR INSERTING A CHEST TUBE:

Prep sponges and antiseptic

Local anesthetic (1% Lidocaine)

22- and 25-gauge needle

10-ml syringe

No. 10 scalpel blade

No. 24–28 chest tube

Kelly clamp

Trocar (optional)

Water seal drainage bottle or system

Rubber connecting tubing

Gauze pads and adhesive tape

# EQUIPMENT

When faced with the need to re-expand a lung, the list of necessary equipment is inversely proportional to the emergency of the situation. Placement of a simple needle into the pleural cavity of a patient with tension pneumothorax usually results in a dramatic clinical improvement. A chest tube can be inserted very rapidly, using only a knife to incise skin and a Kelly clamp to pierce the interspace and insert the tube. If there is sufficient time and the situation does not demand immediate action, it is wise to assemble several other items which will ensure adequate control as well as provide comfort. In addition to material for preping and anesthetizing the skin, a scalpel blade is necessary to make a small skin incision. Many prefer a large chest trocar, which aids tube placement because it includes a sharp point and side arm through which the tube may be advanced with minimal air passage (some tubes are supplied with an internal trocar). Others prefer to pierce the chest wall with a Kelly clamp following local anesthesia.

The chest tube, usually clear silastic, should be of firm construction, size 24 to 28, and have an adequate number of suction holes (3 to 5). Adequate water seal drainage must be assembled in advance so it can be connected immediately after the tube enters the pleural cavity. Finally, large hemostatic Kelly clamps should be present before, during, and after thoracostomy, since chest tubes must be clamped promptly if the closed drainage system becomes disconnected. Chest drainage bottles are discussed in greater detail later.

# TECHNIQUE

Since thoracostomy can be painful, sedate the patient if he is not already experiencing respiratory depression. The appropriate puncture site is the second anterior interspace, beneath the midpoint of the clavicle, particularly in an acute emergency. Prep with a suitable antiseptic and drape with towels. Infiltrate the skin overlying the interspace as well as the intercostal muscles with 1% Lidocaine. While waiting 2–3 minutes (unless there is an acute emergency) for the anesthetic to take effect, make one last check of the tube. If a trocar is to be used, *make certain that the chest tube passes all the way through including the widened hub flange of the tube*! Otherwise, you will be in the unfortunate position of being unable to free the trocar completely once the tube is in place. (If this ever happens cut off the hub rather than remove and replace the tube.) If additional holes are cut in the chest tube, be sure that the most proximal (closest to the skin) is through the radiopaque marking line. Great care should be used in making these holes large enough to be effective but not so large as to weaken the catheter to the point that it will pull apart when it is removed. If the catheter is not marked at intervals to determine its length, tie a suture around it at the exact point on the tube that you would like to be at skin level. Fortunately, modern chest tubes contain multiple appropriately placed holes, radiopaque marking lines and markings to indicate the length of the tube inserted.

When everything is ready, do a thoracentesis in the area to make sure you have a free pleural space. Make a 1.5- to 2-cm stab wound in the skin with a scalpel blade. Insert the Kelly clamp or trocar into the middle of the intercostal space and exert sufficient force to pass through into the pleural sac. Never aim medially; direct the tube slightly outward, thereby avoiding mediastinal injury. Make certain the pleura is pierced before advancing the tube (listen for air). Insert the chest tube 4–6 inches or else to the point where no suction holes remain external to the pleura. Extract the Kelly clamp (or trocar) and connect the chest tube to a length of tubing which leads to a water seal drainage bottle (Fig. 9.1).

In order to secure the chest tube, place one silk suture into the adjacent skin and tie the ends around the tube firmly. Place a heavy purse string in the skin around the tube in preparation for removal of the tube (Fig. 9.2). A light dressing and liberal quantities of adhesive may then be added to ensure stability. Be careful not to bend or kink the tube. Also remember to tape or wire all tube connections carefully in order to avoid air leaks.

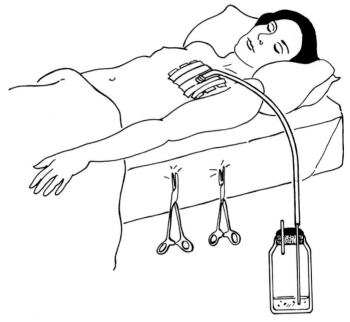

**Figure 9.1.** The tube from the chest connects to the glass tube that is a few centimeters below the water line. Clamps must be kept at the bedside of any patient with functioning chest tubes. In the event of any malfunction, clamp the tube near the chest wall.

## MANAGEMENT OF CHEST DRAINAGE SYSTEMS

The first lesson to be learned is: when in doubt, clamp the chest tube as close to the patient's chest as possible! Any sudden distress or accidental disconnection of the drainage system should be met with this response. Once the patient's pleural cavity is isolated from the room environment, there will be time to ask questions, auscultate, check the lines, replace rubber stoppers, examine the suction source, etc. Therefore, Kelly

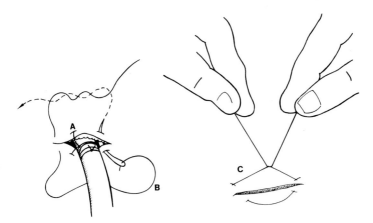

**Figure 9.2.** The chest tube is secured with a heavy suture (A). A heavy purse string suture (B) is placed at the same time but is not tied until the time the chest tube is removed (C).

clamps are to be kept nearby and in plain view (e.g. clipped to the bedsheets) at all times (Fig. 9.1).

Second, remember that there are three types of bottles used in chest cavity drainage: 1) water seal, 2) trap, and 3) control, which may be used in various combinations (Fig. 9.3A). The most important of these is the *water seal* bottle, which serves as a one-way valve, allowing air to be expelled from the thorax but not to return. This is accomplished by connecting the rubber tubing leading from the chest to a glass tube whose tip rests in about 2–4 cm of water (Fig. 9.1). This bottle is always necessary and care should be exercised to assure that the water seal valve is functioning properly. If considerable fluid drainage is expected from the pleural sac (e.g. following pulmonary resection), then a *trap* bottle may be inserted in series but between the patient and the water seal bottle.

The *control* bottle limits the amount of suction that may be applied to the pleural cavity in the following way. There are three holes in the bottle stopper which contain two short glass tubes and one long tube extending almost to the bottom of the

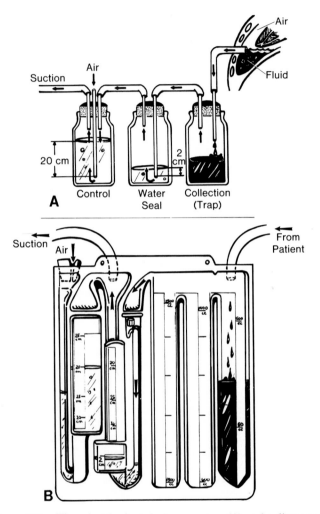

**Figure 9.3.** Three-bottle chest drainage system (A) and a diagram of a clear plastic unistructure device (B) for pleural evacuation.

bottle. One short tube is connected to the water seal bottle and the other to a suction source. The long glass tube remains open to the air but rests beneath a 10- to 20-cm column of water. Whenever the suction source develops a negative pressure greater than the height of the water column, room air will be drawn into the bottle. The use of control bottles are optional but useful for patients with persistent air leaks in whom excessive suction may keep the lung from sealing. These principles have been incorporated into modern unistructure clear plastic devices (Fig. 9.3B).

## REMOVING THE TUBE

Certain details must be remembered to avoid complications when removing a tube. First, determine whether the chest tube is still functioning. In general, the drainage should be <30 ml/day and fluid or air should not be released during a Valsalva maneuver or while coughing. There should be no oscillations for 24 hours. Look at the most recent chest x-ray to make certain that the lung is fully expanded and the tube is ready for removal. If there is more than one chest tube, check the suction bottles and remove the tube that has yielded the least drainage recently. Do not remove two tubes at once! If both are no longer required, remove them on successive days. Don't remove chest tubes late in the day when an x-ray cannot be obtained readily. Otherwise a pneumothorax may remain unnoticed during the night.

An appropriate dose of pain medication prior to removal of the chest tube will make the procedure less painful. Assemble in advance a heavy gauze dressing on which is layered either antibiotic ointment or Vaseline gauze. This helps to assure an air-tight seal at the tube site. Also have plenty of adhesive tape on hand. Start by clamping the tube to interrupt all suction. Remove the overlying dressing and cut any retaining sutures. Twist the tube to dislodge any adherent lung tissue inside (otherwise the lung may be injured when the tube is removed). If a purse-string suture was placed at the time of the chest tube insertion, snug this around the tube site. Otherwise place the already prepared dressing over the tube entrance site, ask the patient to take two deep breaths, and remove the tube quickly at the end of the second expiration (air might be sucked in if the tube is removed during inspiration). Another technique is to pull the tube while the patient is doing a Valsalva. Maintain pressure on the dressing and fix it well with strips of wide adhesive tape. A small dressing may be substituted 48 hours later. Always obtain a chest x-ray 1–2 hours after removing a tube to make certain that the lung remains expanded. If the patient is in distress, obtain the chest x-ray immediately. Recurrent pneumothorax must be treated by prompt tube reinsertion (usually using another site).

## COMPLICATIONS

A number of complications which occur following thoracentesis may also result from thoracostomy, e.g. hemorrhage from an injured intercostal artery. However, in addition, there are sequelae quite specific to thoracostomy such as mediastinal trauma and extra-pleural placement of the tube following incomplete entry of the pleural space. Patients with recurrent pneumothorax should not have tubes placed directly over a previous thoracostomy site since pulmonary adhesions are common and the tube may be plunged directly into the lung parenchyma. Pain often follows insertion of a chest tube and medication may be required for 2–3 days. Intercostal nerve block occasionally becomes necessary as well.

Subcutaneous emphysema may develop in the surrounding chest wall if the tube becomes partially occluded, the last hole is outside the pleural space, or there is insufficient suction to remove the pleural air. Subcutaneous emphysema is rarely a serious development but does call for close examination and adjustment of the chest suction apparatus.

Infection can occur around the tube site if there is an empyema or if the tube is placed through one of the original traumatic chest openings. This possibility can be minimized by using careful technique and placing the chest tube through a new stab wound under controlled conditions.

## Selected References for Further Reading

1. Adkins, P. C. Preoperative and postoperative care of the thoracic surgery patients. In *Surgical Diseases of the Chest*, edited by B. Blades. C.V. Mosby, St. Louis, 1961, pp. 54–68.
2. Langston, H. T., Pantone, A. M., and Melamed, M. *The Postoperative Chest*. Charles C Thomas, Springfield, Ill., 1958.
3. Lindskog, G. E. and Halasz, N. A. Spontaneous pneumothorax. *Arch. Surg. (Chicago) 75:* 693–698, 1957.
4. Spencer, F. C. Treatment of chest injuries. *Curr. Probl. Surg.* 1–36, 1964.
5. Steier, M., Ching, N., Bonfils, E., and Nealon, T. F. Pneumothorax complicating continuous ventilatory support. *J. Thorac. Cardiovasc. Surg. 67:* 17–23, 1974.
6. Timmis, H. H., Virgilio, R., and McClenathan, J. E. Spontaneous pneumothorax. *Amer. J. Surg. 110:* 929–934, 1965.
7. Woods, J. M. Experiences with pneumothorax in a general hospital. *Surg. Gynec. Obstet. 121:* 1315–1324, 1965.

## TEN

# Resuscitation

Cardiopulmonary resuscitation (CPR) demands an organized team effort. There is just too much to do all at once for any one person to be consistently successful. On the other hand, if too much help is present, the result may be chaos and failure! Any health professional might find himself in the unexpected position of initiating or assisting a resuscitation attempt. Only a physician may carry out advanced life support, but the techniques of basic life support can be mastered by all citizens. This chapter considers some of the measures which may be used in the event of cardiac or pulmonary arrest. They are listed in approximate chronologic order. Because time is so very important, it is essential that priorities be established so that the response is quick and automatic.

1. *Confirm Diagnosis.* Cardiac arrest is usually discovered by someone other than a physician, who has been taught to call for help (each hospital will have a special code, e.g. Code Blue, Code 99, etc.) whenever there is doubt about the patient's medical stability. The first physician to arrive should determine quickly what has happened to the patient and which vital functions have ceased. This does not mean that resuscitative efforts must be withheld until a precise diagnosis has been made, but there must be a presumption of what has taken place moments before. First, try to awaken the patient with a loud voice and by shaking the patient. A rapid assessment can be made by feeling for the carotid or femoral pulse with one hand while checking for respiratory function with the other (place hand on the chest wall or over the patient's mouth).

Look at the pupils to get an idea of how long the patient has been without heart action (dilation begins 45 seconds after the heart stops and is complete after 2 minutes).

2. *Make a Decision to Resuscitate.* The first physician on the scene must decide whether to institute resuscitation or not. Once underway, all who arrive afterward are likely to pitch in. Considerable time might elapse before any thought is given to the result of resuscitation. If the patient's pupils are already fixed and dilated and there is indication that death occurred several minutes prior to this discovery, then there is just cause for omitting resuscitation. Remember that irreversible brain damage occurs in 4–6 minutes. Therefore, cerebral oxygenation must begin within this time period or the patient can be left with permanent central nervous system injury. There is little justification for attempting to revive a terminal cancer patient. Although advanced medical technology permits us to maintain vital functions almost indefinitely, even this possibility does not justify senseless resuscitation.

3. *Call for Help.* Having decided to go ahead, make certain that assistance is on the way. Calling a "code" to recruit more people is essential. This will mean at least one other physician and preferably two. If a representative of the anesthesia department is available, he should be among the first to be summoned, so that he might establish and maintain an adequate airway.

The nurse must also have assistance. If she is alone in the middle of the night, then help must be provided by the supervisor or a nurse from a nearby ward. There should always be a minimum of two nurses, one to remain in the patient's room and assist with drug administration, and another to run for additional medication and equipment. A "crash cart" previously stocked with essential drugs, fluids, and equipment should be made available at the scene of the CPR. A clerk or nurse should record the events in accurate chronological order, noting the exact time that each drug was given or procedure accomplished. Finally, an electrocardiogram must be obtained as quickly as possible.

4. *Establish an Airway.* The aforementioned activities should

require but a few seconds since they can largely be carried out simultaneously. The first therapeutic action to be taken is establishment of an airway and initiation of adequate respiratory exchange. A mistake which is often made is to commence cardiac massage while another physician struggles to insert an endotracheal tube as the patient's head bobs with each sternal compression. Assisted circulation is of no value whatever in the absence of adequate respiratory exchange. Therefore, the airway definitely takes precedence!

Cardic arrest can be produced by airway blockage alone. The "restaurant coronary" follows aspiration of a piece of solid food into the larynx. The diagnosis is made by any of the symptoms or signs listed in Table 10.1. The immediate treatment is four sharp blows to the midback followed by a rapid intraoral sweep of the finger to remove the blockage. If this is not successful, a Heimlich Maneuver should be done. This maneuver is accomplished by grabbing the patient around the lower chest in a bear hug and giving a quick forceful squeeze which will often dislodge a laryngeal obstruction.

Endotracheal intubation is the fastest and surest means for

**Table 10.1. First Aid for Choking (from American Heart Association)**

| Conscious Victim | Unconscious Victim |
| --- | --- |
| 1. If the victim gives the *universal sign* for choking (open hand spread across the anterior neck) but *can* speak, cough and/or breathe, do not interfere. | 1. Open airway and try to ventilate |
| 2. If the victim *cannot* speak, cough or breathe, give 4 quick back blows with the heel of the hand. | 2. If unsuccessful, give 4 quick back blows with the heel of the hand. |
| 3. If unsuccessful, give 4 upward abdominal thrusts or 4 backward chest thrusts (about CPR site). | 3. If unsuccessful, give 4 abdominal or chest thrusts |
| 4. Repeat above sequence. Be persistent. Continue uninterrupted until advanced life support is available. | 4. If unsuccessful, try finger probe. Repeat above sequence. Be persistent. Continue uninterrupted until advanced life support is available. |

achieving satisfactory ventilation, but it requires skill and experience (Figs. 10.1 and 10.2). If you are not experienced, then insert an oropharyngeal airway and apply mouth-to-mouth or Ambu respiration until someone more capable arrives to insert a tube (Fig. 10.3). Whenever the situation is desperate, the airway must be established in the neck by coniotomy (see Chapter Twelve).

5. *External Cardiac Massage.* Since the introduction of assisted circulation by sternal compression, open or internal cardiac massage is rarely used and only then under special conditions (e.g. if chest is already open or in the presence of severe thoracic trauma such as crushed chest, cardiac tamponade, or cardiac wounds). Except for the severely emphysematous patient with an unyielding rib cage, force properly applied to the mid-lower

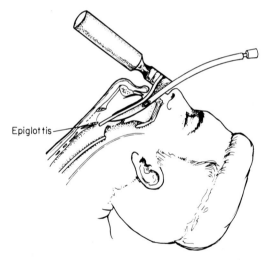

Epiglottis

**Figure 10.1.** Endotracheal intubation is the fastest and surest means of achieving a satisfactory airway. Infants should not be hyperextended since the vocal cords can be seen better in neutral position. Likewise pressure on the back of an infant's tongue will move the epiglottis out of the way.

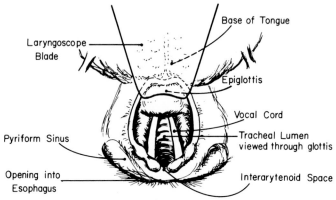

**Figure 10.2.**   Intraoral view of trachea during intubation.

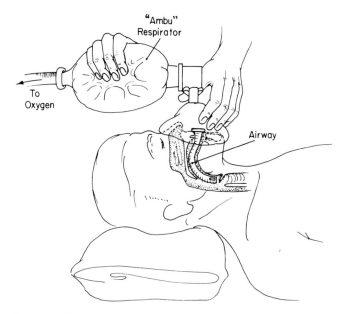

**Figure 10.3.**   Adequate temporary breathing support may be achieved with an oral airway and Ambu respirator.

sternum will produce a systolic pressure of 90–110 mm Hg with a mean of 40–50 mm Hg. With the patient supine, and on a flat hard surface (e.g. a backboard or on the floor), kneel by the patient. Place the heel of your hand on the lower one-third of the sternum (not on xyphoid process). Sharply depress the sternum 3–5 cm using both hands, one over the other. Interlock and curl the fingers such that the entire force is delivered through the heel of the hand in contact with the sternum. Great caution must be taken to remain in the midline with each and every stroke (Fig. 10.4). If the hand strays lateral to the sternum, then the heart will receive inadequate compression force and there will be risk of fractured ribs whose tips might be driven into the lung or liver. Maintain a compression rate of 60/minute. Keep the sternum compressed for one-half the cycle. After pushing the sternum down, hold it down for a moment and then release so that the compression phase is as long as the release phase. There should be no pause in this rhythm (unless one is performing CPR unassisted). Ventilation should be coordinated such that the lungs are inflated in between every 4th and 5th external cardiac massage without a break in the rhythm. The accepted sequence for unassisted CPR is 2 breaths followed by 15 external cardiac massages at

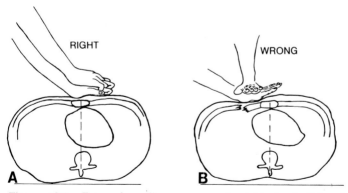

**Figure 10.4.** External cardiac massage: A, right—heel of hand placed in midline; B, wrong—hand has strayed lateral to base of sternum.

a rate of 72/min. One useful method for monitoring the effectiveness of external cardiac massage is to apply a sphygmomanometer to one arm and inflate it to 90 mm Hg. Each deflection of the needle will then represent a satisfactory stroke while absence of deflection calls for additional force. Don't use the carotid artery to monitor compression, since digital pressure might further compromise an already marginal blood flow to the brain.

Infants require very little force for the maintenance of effective circulation. This can be accomplished by compressing the sternum with 2 fingers at a rate of 100/minute while holding one hand behind the infant.

6. *Establish Access to the Circulation.* If an intravenous infusion is not already functioning, one must be started at once since most of the treatment which follows depends on the ability to inject a variety of drugs directly into the circulation. Following arrest, efforts to insert a needle percutaneously usually fail because there is little or no venous pressure. Rather than waste valuable time proceed with a cutdown (Chapter Four), using the greater saphenous vein in the ankle. Subclavian or femoral vein puncture is another possible route to the venous circulation.

7. *Establish a Diagnosis.* Once sufficient help is assembled, an airway provided, circulation assisted, and an intravenous route obtained, the general speed of activity can be reduced as the second phase of resuscitation begins. Efforts are now turned to a study of the probable cause of arrest and a well-timed and coordinated attempt to re-establish cardiac activity. If the cause of arrest was hypoxia, then the measures performed thus far might result in resumption of a normal rhythm and blood pressure. Regardless of the cause, however, an electrocardiogram is essential, since all subsequent therapy depends on a precise knowledge of the cardiac rhythm.

8. *Treat Acidosis.* Regardless of the cause, inadequate circulation leads to severe tissue acidosis which must be treated aggressively. Sodium bicarbonate can be started as soon as an intravenous line is established. Adult cardiac arrest victims should receive 2 ampules (44.6–50 mEq each) or its equivalent

initially. Blood gas measurements should be used to guide subsequent bicarbonate administrations; otherwise, if they are not available, give one ampule every 10–15 minutes. Units of 500 ml containing 297 mEq of sodium bicarbonate are available which can be infused continuously, making the treatment of acidosis easier.

9. *Defibrillation.* If the electrocardiogram demonstrates ventricular fibrillation or ventricular tachycardia, reversion to sinus rhythm requires the immediate use of a defibrillating current. Most devices designed for this purpose require two external paddles well coated with conductive cream applied to the chest wall (one at the cardiac apex and the other at the cardiac base). Operation of the defibrillator units will vary somewhat but 100–400 watt-seconds of direct current are ordinarily sufficient to interrupt fibrillatory rhythm. Most authorities recommend starting low and adding power if necessary, but there is no danger in starting with the maximum and simply repeating it if the first shock is ineffective. If 3 or 4 shocks in quick succession fail to work, the heart is probably hypoxic and will require 2–3 minutes more CPR before defibrillation can be tried again. As an added safeguard against personal injury, rubber gloves should be worn by the person holding the paddles on the chest wall and *no one should be in direct contact with the patient or the bed at the moment of impulse* (most ECG machines must be disconnected also).

10. *Cardiac Stimulation.* If the electrocardiogram demonstrates cardiac asystole, then inaugurate cardiac rhythm by giving epinephrine chloride (0.5 mg diluted with 8–10 ml of saline) into a central vein or directly into the vertricle. Be careful to inject the drug into the chamber rather than into the ventricular wall or the resulting irritable focus might produce fibrillation. The intracardiac injection can be delivered via the subcostal route (Chapter Eight). A 20-gauge/3-inch needle is inserted, aiming toward the back of the patient's left shoulder. Advance the needle while aspirating. Immediately on drawing blood, inject the drug and quickly remove the needle. Alternatively, the apex may be punctured by putting the needle in below the left breast in the mid-clavicular line, going over the

rib and aiming for the right shoulder. *All of these routes are dangerous and should be used only if the heart is in standstill and there is no IV route.*

*11. Administer Other Medication as Indicated.* Dopamine (0.5–4 mg/minute) may be helpful in temporarily supporting the blood pressure after normal rhythm has resumed. Calcium chloride (1 gm) may strengthen the force of heart contractions. For premature ventricular or tachycardia contractions, intravenous Lidocaine (50 mg intravenously and then 1–4 mg/minute as a slow infusion) is extremely effective in suppressing the irritability of the heart and preventing recurrent fibrillation.

12. *Monitor the Patient!* The incidence of recurrent arrest after successful resuscitation is extremely high. Therefore, a cardiac monitor and special nursing care are absolutely essential, particularly during the first 24 hours following arrest.

In summary, resuscitation may either be coordinated or chaotic. Success is not exclusively associated with the former, but rarely accompanies the latter. Although each clinical circumstance differs, performance of these twelve therapeutic steps may result in success. Throughout the period of resuscitation, whether it be 30 seconds or 30 minutes, one person (usually the senior physician in attendance or the doctor most closely involved in the patient's care) must serve as leader and direct the course of action according to the electrocardiographic findings and the patient's response. There is no place for simultaneous conflicting treatment decisions by several different physicians. Similarly, it is the role of one man to determine when, in the face of persistent failure, further efforts should be made. This is always a difficult decision since there are no rules which define the maximum amount of time which should be devoted to cardiac resuscitation. Absence of a satisfactory cardiac response in the face of progressive pupillary dilation usually points to failure.

### Selected References for Further Reading

1. Jude, J. R., Kouwenhoven, W. B., and Knickerbocker, G. G. External cardiac massage. *Monogr. Surg. Sci. 1:* 59–117, 1964.

2. Messer, J. V. Current concepts: cardiac arrest. *New Eng. J. Med. 275:* 35–39, 1966.
3. Stephenson, H. E. *Cardiac Arrest and Resuscitation*, 2nd Ed. C. V. Mosby, St. Louis, 1964.
4. Vanway, C. W., III and Buerk, C. A. Cardiopulmonary resuscitation. In *Surgical Skills in Patient Care.* C. V. Mosby, St. Louis, 1978, pp. 158–164.

## ELEVEN

# The Electrocardiogram

One of the more frequently performed clinical procedures is the electrocardiogram. The electrocardiogram (ECG or EKG) is a graphic recording of the electrical potentials produced in association with the heartbeat. Pacemaker cells in the heart (S-A Node) produce electrical impulses which are carried by the conduction system to the myocardium where this impulse produces depolarization and subsequent contraction of the myocardium. Depolarization and repolarization of the myocardium produce weak electric currents that spread throughout the body. By applying electrodes to various positions of the body and connecting these electrodes to an electrocardiographic apparatus, the electrocardiogram is produced. The amplified signal can be recorded permanently on paper (the ECG) or it can appear on a cardioscope as an electrographic pattern on a florescent screen which is of particular value in the constant electrographic observation of the patient.

The electrocardiogram is an analog representation of cardiac electrical activity and is not the sine qua non for the diagnosis of heart disease. Patients with an organic heart disorder may demonstrate a normal electrocardiogram while a perfectly normal individual may show nonspecific electrocardiographic abnormalities. The electrocardiogram, therefore, must be interpreted in the context of clinical findings.

## EQUIPMENT

There are many varieties of electrocardiographic machines and cardioscopes. In recent years, ECG tracings can be transmitted by telephone to data centers where they are interpreted by sophisticated computers, a probable diagnosis made, and recommendations for further investigation or treatment transmitted back to the source. It behooves the health professional to study the individual machine in depth so that he has an understanding of the capabilities of his particular apparatus. Moreover, an improperly performed electrocardiogram may lead to misinformation or perhaps no information at all. Therefore, proper application of the electrodes and recording of the impulses is of paramount importance. This chapter deals with the general principles for obtaining a standard electrocardiogram. Interpretive discussions may be found in specialized texts.

## TECHNIQUE

To insure a technically acceptable tracing without artifacts, the patient should lie in a comfortable bed or on an examining table large enough to support his entire body. He should be completely relaxed. The entire procedure is explained to the patient in order to relieve the fear and anxiety associated with attachment to a machine.

Electrodes are applied to the right arm (white electrode), the left arm (black electrode), the right leg (green electrode), and the left leg (red electrode). Proper skin contact is obtained by using electrode paste in contact with skin. The right leg electrode serves as a ground wire and plays no role in the production of the electrical pattern. If the machine does not have this feature, it may be necessary to run a ground wire from the bed or the machine to an appropriate ground (water pipe or steam pipe) to eliminate electrical interference (Fig. 11.1).

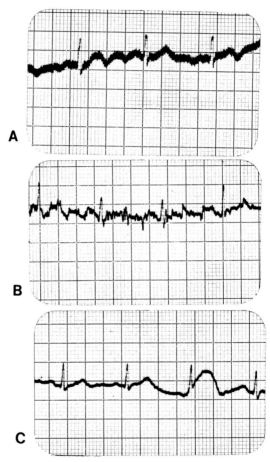

**Figure 11.1.** Effect of alternating current interference (A) muscle twitching (B), and poor contact (C).

The electrical potential as recorded from any single extremity will be the same no matter where the electrode is placed on the extremity. The electrodes are usually applied just above the wrists and ankles. If an extremity has been amputated, the electrode can be applied to the stump. If the patient has extensive burns, needle electrodes may be used. Patients with an uncontrollable tremor will provide satisfactory recordings if electrodes are attached to the proximal arm or leg.

The bipolar leads represent a difference in electrical potential between two selected sites.

Standard Lead 1 is the difference in potential between the left arm and right arm (LA-RA).

Standard Lead 2 is the difference in potential between the left leg and right arm (LL-RA)

Standard Lead 3 is the difference in potential between the left leg and the left arm (LL-LA).

These may be obtained by turning the selector dial to I, II, and III (Fig. 11.2).

All modern electrocardiogram devices are constructed so that augmented extremity leads may be taken with the same hookup as used for standard leads, simply by turning the selector dial to aVR, aVL, and aVF (Fig. 11.2). These unipolar leads record all the electrical events of the entire cardiac cycle as viewed from the selected lead site.

Unipolar chest leads are recorded by applying the chest lead and its electrode (usually in the form of a suction cup) to any desired position on the chest and turning the selector dial to the V lead position (Fig. 11.2). Multiple chest leads are taken by changing the position of the chest electrodes (Fig. 11.3). Unipolar esophageal leads are taken by attaching the esophageal lead to the chest lead and turning the selector dial to the V lead position.

Although many electrocardiographic machines have six different chest leads (individual electrodes and wires making it possible to take simultaneous chest leads), some of the machines still require that the chest electrode be applied in a sequential fashion to the desired chest positions producing multiple unipolar chest leads (Fig. 11.3). The standard precordial positions recommended by the American Heart Association are as follows:

$V_1$ Fourth intercostal space at the right sternal border

$V_2$ Fourth intercostal space at the left sternal border

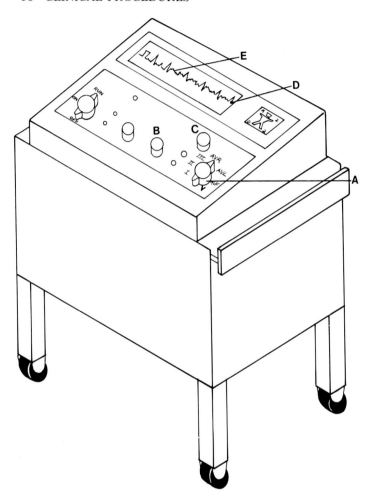

**Figure 11.2.** Diagram of control panel of electrocardiographic machine showing the lead selector (A), standardization button (B), standardization gain knob (C), writing pen (D), and electrocardiogram paper (E).

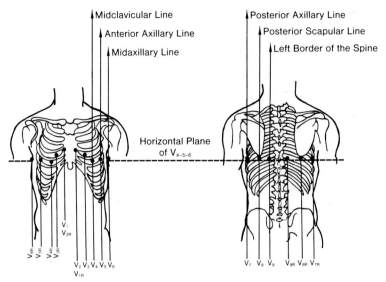

**Figure 11.3.**  Locations of unipolar precordial leads.

$V_3$  Equal distance between $V_2$ and $V_4$

$V_4$  Fifth intercostal space in the left midclavicular line (all subsequent leads $V_5$–$V_9$ are taken in the same horizontal plane as $V_4$)

$V_5$  Anterior axillary line

$V_6$  Midaxillary line

$V_7$  Posterior axillary line (optional)

$V_8$  Posterior scapular line (optional)

$V_9$  Left border of the spine (optional)

Right unipolar precordial leads ($V_{2R}$–$V_{9R}$) are taken on the right side of the chest in the same relative locations as the left sided leads $V_{3-9}$ with $V_{2R}$ the same as $V_1$ (Fig. 11.3). Additional leads can be taken, but this is not standard practice.

The routine electrocardiogram consists of 12 leads: I, II, III, aVR, aVL, aVF, and $V_1$–$V_6$. The standard international marking system is shown on the sample tracings in Fig. 11.4. Often, a standard lead II is taken for a longer period of time to identify an arrhythmia. It may be taken as a "rhythm strip" on a standard electrocardiogram or it may be recorded from time to time as a permanent recording of a cardioscope.

Before and after running each twelve lead electrocardiogram or rhythm strip, a standardization signal should be placed on the electrocardiogram (Fig. 11.4). The machine must be properly standardized so that one millivolt will produce a deflection of 1 cm (10 small boxes). Incorrect standardization produces inaccurate voltage and faulty interpretation. Over standardization increases the voltage of the complexes and understandardization decreases the voltage of the complexes.

Muscular activity by the patient must be held to a minimum (Fig. 11.1B). Poor contact between the skin and the electrode can result in a poor record (Fig. 11.1C). The patient and the machine must be properly grounded to avoid alternating current interference (Fig. 11.1A).

A standard electrocardiogram is a noninvasive procedure and may, therefore, easily be practiced on volunteers (perhaps your colleague). The paper used for recording is relatively inexpensive and medical personnel can practice this procedure until they become proficient without great expense. Then, when an electrocardiogram is required, it can be performed with proficiency. The electrocardiogram is of particular value in the following clinical conditions:

1. Atrial and ventricular hypertrophy
2. Myocardial infarction
3. Arrhythmia
4. Pericarditis
5. Systemic diseases which affect the heart
6. Effect of cardiac drugs and other drugs used for other conditions
7. Electrolyte disturbances such as potassium abnormalities

While other more sophisticated methods of evaluating cardiac function are available (vector cardiograms, cardiac catheteri-

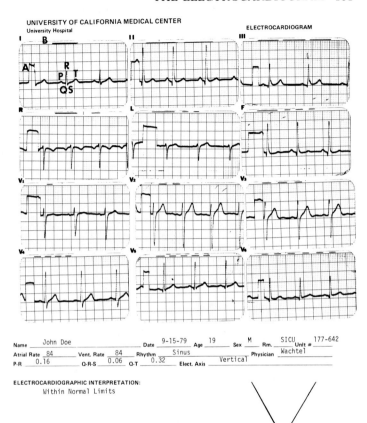

Name ___John Doe___   Date ___9-15-79___  Age ___19___  Sex ___M___  Rm. ___SICU___ Unit # ___177-642___

Atrial Rate ___84___   Vent. Rate ___84___  Rhythm ___Sinus___   Physician ___Wachtel___

P-R ___0.16___   Q-R-S ___0.06___  Q-T ___0.32___  Elect. Axis ___Vertical___

ELECTROCARDIOGRAPHIC INTERPRETATION:
    Within Normal Limits

**Figure 11.4.** Standard 12 lead ECG with standardization signal (A) international marking code (B) and representative normal pattern for each lead.

zation, echo cardiograms, radiocardiograms, etc.), the standard 12 lead electrocardiogram and the continuous cardioscopic monitoring remain the mainstay of cardiac evaluation.

### Selected References for Further Reading

1. Beckwith, J. R. *Grant's Clinical Electrocardiography*, 2nd Ed. McGraw-Hill Book Co., New York, 1970.
2. Burch, G. E. and Winsor, T. *A Primer of Electrocardiography*. Lea & Febiger, Philadelphia, 1972.
3. Chung, E. K. *Electrocardiography*. Harper & Row, Hagerstown, Md., 1974.
4. Cooksey, J. D., Dunn, M., and Massie, E.: *Clinical Vectorcardiography and Electrocardiography*, 2nd Ed. Yearbook Medical Publishers Inc., Chicago, 1977.
5. Goldman, M. J. *Principles of Clinical Electrocardiography*. Lang Medical Publications, Los Altos, Ca., 1962, pp. 1–16.
6. Hohn, A. R. *Basic Pediatric Electrocardiography*. Medcom Press, New York, 1974.
7. Krupp, M. A., Sweet, N. J., and Jawetzen Armstrong, C. D. Cardiography. In *Physicians Handbook*. Lang Medical Publishers, Los Altos, Ca., 1962, pp. 64–89.
8. Silverman, M. E. and Silverman, B. D. The diagnostic capabilities and limitations of the electrocardiogram. In *The Heart*, Edited by J. W. Hurst. McGraw-Hill Book Co., New York, 1979.

# TWELVE

# Tracheostomy

Tracheostomy is certainly not a minor clinical procedure. On the contrary, experienced surgeons gain renewed respect for the operation each time they must perform it rapidly under less than ideal circumstances. One might then consider a discussion of tracheostomy inappropriate for this volume. However, because students are frequently asked to assist during its performance, as well as to participate in the postoperative care of the tracheal stoma, consideration of this subject seems fully justified. In fact, the importance of tracheostomy in the maintenance of a satisfactory airway makes it a topic of urgent concern for all health professionals.

## HISTORY

Tracheostomy was first performed by Asklepiades, a first century Roman physician, who recognized its value for patients with diphtheria. During the second century, Antyllus recognized the difference between high tracheal obstruction and inflammatory disease of the lung noting that tracheostomy was of benefit only in the first instance. Many similar reports appeared during subsequent centuries and numerous paintings depicted the performance of tracheostomy as a means of reviving victims of drowning. The widespread European diphtheria epidemics of the 18th and 19th centuries further established the usefulness and popularity of this procedure.

Early American physicians were more reluctant to admit the benefits of tracheostomy. The team of physicians caring for George Washington during his final illness, a severe case of tracheobronchitis, rejected the operation, perhaps because it was suggested by their youngest member.

Tracheostomy eventually achieved widespread popularity during the 19th and early 20th centuries. Its use today has been tempered somewhat because there are faster methods of securing an emergency airway (e.g. endotracheal intubation) and the procedure in some clinical situations, such as severe thermal injury, is often associated with serious complications. Nevertheless, the benefits of tracheostomy in the event of facial fractures, severe chest injury, head and neck surgery, and long-term respiratory support assures its essential role in medical practice.

# EQUIPMENT

Tracheostomy instrument sets usually include many more instruments than are actually necessary. However, a number of items are particularly important and their presence deserves confirmation before starting. Almost any scalpel blade will be satisfactory for the skin incision, but only a small delicate blade (e.g. No. 15 or 11 Bard Parker or No. 44 Beaver) is necessary for fenestrating the trachea. Two medium-sized retractors (e.g. Army-Navy) must be available to provide exposure of the trachea. A smaller retractor (e.g. Cushing vein retractor) is helpful if a low-lying thyroid isthmus must be pulled upward to expose the tracheal rings. At least one and preferably two hooks must be present for holding the trachea while it is opened. A three-bladed spreader may also be helpful for enlarging the tracheal stoma to facilitate tube insertion, but great care must be taken to prevent the fracturing of cartilages with this device. Finally, make certain that a reasonable assortment of tracheostomy tubes are nearby (Nos. 5–9 for adults, Nos. 2–5 for infants and children.

Tracheostomy tubes are constructed of rubber, plastic, or

stainless steel. The first two are disposable and have the added advantage of incorporating inflatable cuffs which are essential whenever mechanically assisted respiration is applied. Cuffs may also be applied to metal tubes, but there is a danger of balloon dislodgement and aspiration unless a strong adhesive is used. The cuffs should be of the low pressure, large volume variety.

## TECHNIQUE

Fortunately, the days of the bedside tracheostomy under flashlight illumination are past. In the event of apnea requiring immediate access to the trachea, endotracheal intubation or incision of the cricothyroid ligament (coniotomy) are the procedures of choice (Fig. 12.1). Under most other conditions, tracheostomy should be performed in a surgical environment or the complication rate will be intolerably frequent. This means a brightly illuminated and well supplied operating room! A standby anesthetist may also be helpful and necessary if an endotracheal tube should be passed prior to tracheostomy.

Begin by positioning the patient with a sheet roll under his shoulders so that the head is fully extended (Fig. 12.2). If the patient is alert, be free with explanatory comments since tracheostomy candidates are often near panic as the procedure begins. Prep the entire neck, drape the patient, and infiltrate the skin over the incision site with 1% Lidocaine.

Opinions vary regarding the best incision for tracheostomy. Actually, any controversy between the proponents of the vertical and horizontal incision is unnecessary since each method has its inherent advantages and disadvantages and there is no "best" way. The vertical incision is safest, since all dissection is performed in the midline away from major vessels and quickest, since the trachea can be more easily exposed. The transverse incision, on the other hand, is slightly more difficult and requires an experienced operator with an excellent assistant to provide exposure, but has definite cosmetic advantages in that the scar, although no smaller than the following vertical inci-

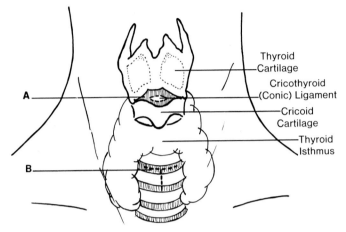

Thyroid
Cartilage

Cricothyroid
(Conic) Ligament

Cricoid
Cartilage

Thyroid
Isthmus

A

B

**Figure 12.1.** In the event of an emergency requiring an immediate airway (e.g. cyanosis following aspiration), the trachea may be entered through the cricothyroid ligament (A). Elective tracheostomy should be performed beneath the thyroid isthmus (third or fourth tracheal ring) (B).

sion, is usually less noticeable, since it lies in the direction of the natural skin crease. Subsequent transverse scar revision is also more easily carried out. Vertical incisions should extend from the thyroid cartilage to above the sternal notch (3–6 cm, depending on the size of the patient). Transverse incisions should be made in a skin crease half-way between these two landmarks. Divide not only the skin, but also the subcutaneous tissue and platysma muscle. Stop at this point and ligate or cauterize any vigorously bleeding superficial vessels. Now ask your assistant to retract the wound edges with two retractors. Taking tissue forceps in one hand and dissecting scissors in the other, separate the strap muscles using longitudinal spreading motions (Fig. 12.3). Further dissection should be limited strictly to the midline, and the best way of staying there is to stop periodically and *palpate the trachea with a fingertip.* As each muscular layer is divided, the assistant should place the retrac-

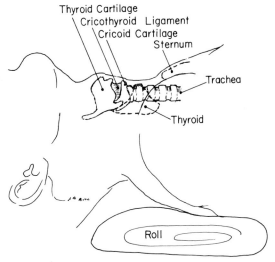

**Figure 12.2.** Place a sheet roll beneath the shoulders in order to hyperextend the neck prior to tracheostomy.

tor blades deeper and expose the next layer. The trachea will soon come into view, hopefully with little or no bleeding. Major hemorrhage usually appears after straying from midline and damaging the internal jugular vein or one of its branches.

Watch carefully for the thyroid isthmus which firmly overlies the first and second tracheal rings. Occasionally, it lies in a lower position and must be clamped, divided, and tied. More commonly, once the tracheal rings are in view, the inferior edge of the isthmus can be drawn superiorly by a small vein retractor. Now clear the last few strands of connective tissue off the anterior surface and sides of the trachea and select a stoma site, usually the third or fourth ring. If the wound is dry and the trachea well exposed, grasp a ring with one or two hooks above and below the fenestration site. Ask your assistant to remove the wound retractors since the trachea can now be very satisfactorily exposed by traction.

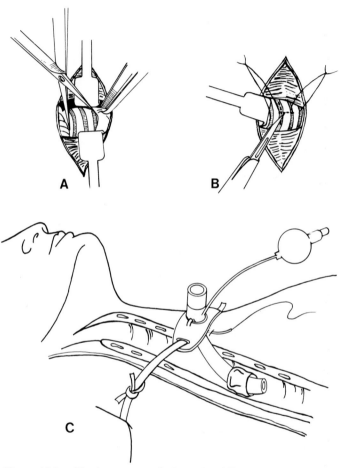

**Figure 12.3.** Tracheostomy technique: A, while an assistant retracts, expose the trachea using forceps and dissecting scissors. Remain in midline and avoid injury to the thyroid isthmus. B, retract the isthmus superiorly, grasp the trachea with a hook, and incise between the second and third rings. Always place guide sutures around the 2nd and 4th cartilaginous rings so that the tracheostomy tube that is

Topical anesthetic (2–3 ml of 2% Pontocaine) may be instilled into the trachea at this point to depress the cough reflex. If an endotracheal tube is in place, warn the anesthesiologist so that he may deflate the balloon before the trachea is incised. Make one last check for bleeding points since they will be inaccessible once the tracheostomy tube is in place. Using a small blade, cut a transverse incision in the tracheal wall between two tracheal rings. A T-shaped incision is made by cutting the next lower cartilaginous ring in the midline. Insert guide sutures through the trachea above and below the incision. Tie them well outside the skin so that they can be removed easily at some later date.

Finally, lubricate the tip of the tracheostomy tube and insert it into the tracheal lumen. If it does not enter easily, use the three-bladed spreader to hold the tracheal incision open. Once the tube is in place, place a hand over the orifice to be certain that air is being expelled through it. Remove all hooks and retractors and promptly secure the tube with cloth ties around the neck or by suturing the tube to the skin. *Never let go of the tube until it is tied in place or it may be coughed out.* Finish by aspirating any blood which might have drained into the trachea from the wound. A few skin sutures may be needed but remember that, if the wound is closed too tightly about the tube, subcutaneous emphysema may develop.

## MAINTENANCE

There are two essential features of proper tracheostomy care: provision of humidity and removal of secretions. Remember that a tracheostomy bypasses the nasal passages and pharynx where humidification normally takes place. Many nebulizers are now available which supply warm humidified air (which

---

accidentally removed can be easily replaced. C, always tie the tracheostomy tube securely in place so it will not be inadvertently coughed out. Cuffed tube pressures will be monitored frequently and the cuff deflated periodically.

is preferable to cold air since it holds more moisture). Another method of providing moisture to the trachea and lower respiratory passages is to drip normal saline very slowly into the tracheostomy stoma.

Aspiration of secretions not only becomes easier following tracheostomy, but also more important since patients lose their ability to cough effectively as soon as they become unable to raise endobronchial pressure behind the closed glottis. Therefore, even though tracheostomy patients appear to be coughing adequately, they are indeed less capable of expelling their own secretions than a person with an intact trachea. Endotracheal suction should be carried out every 30–60 minutes when secretions are profuse. Keep a suction machine, sterile plastic gloves, and several disposable plastic suction catheters by the bedside so that secretions can be removed each time that the patient is seen by a nurse or physician. Do not apply suction for excessive periods of time or the patient will become hypoxic. One excellent precaution is to *hold your own breath* while suction is applied.

Tracheostomy tubes should not be changed during the first 48 hours in order to permit a tract to form. Otherwise, replacement may be difficult. If the tube is inadvertently coughed out during the first 2 days, the patient might become cyanotic following tracheal stomal recession beneath the tissue planes. Gentle traction on the guide sutures will assist replacement of the tracheostomy tube. A laryngoscope with an infant blade is useful for reinserting any tracheostomy tube, but most particularly for children. The first elective tube change should be performed with adequate light, one assistant, and either a tracheostomy set or a laryngoscope nearby.

Day-to-day care of tracheostomy tubes should include removal of the inner cannula two or three times daily for cleaning and removal of inspissated secretions. Many modern plastic tubes do not have inner cannulae and require periodic changes to clean them. Patients complaining of difficulty breathing should have their tube removed promptly. Sudden relief usually means the tube was plugged. If respiratory distress continues, a bronchoscope should be inserted into the stoma, since plugs of inspissated secretions often collect just below the end of the tube.

## COMPLICATIONS

Many studies have shown that the complication rate following tracheostomy is as high as 30%. One report noted that 65% of patients with long-term tracheostomy experienced at least one complication. These data further support the view that tracheostomy is not a minor procedure.

Operative complications are usually a result of poor lighting and inadequate exposure. Hemorrhage follows injury to the thyroid isthmus or major vessels of the neck. The recurrent nerve may be damaged if the dissection strays into the tissue lateral to the trachea. Both accidents can be avoided by operating carefully and remaining in midline. If the isthmus obstructs access to the trachea or is inadvertently injured, then it should be dissected free of the trachea, doubly clamped, divided, and ligated with 3-0 catgut. Esophageal perforation may result from careless entry into the trachea. Remember that the esophagus lies adherent to the back wall of the trachea. Pneumothorax may occur when tracheostomy is performed in children since the pleural dome lies extremely close to the trachea.

Early postoperative complications include subcutaneous emphysema following excessively tight skin closure around the tube. Also, respiratory arrest and death may result from either dislodgement of cannula or false passage of the tube into the mediastinum rather than the tracheal lumen. Therefore, when changing tubes, always be certain that the tube lies within the trachea and is tied in place securely before leaving the patient.

Late complications are usually related to inadequate care and include stenosis, cannula obstruction, and purulent tracheitis. Tracheal stenosis may follow the prolonged use of a cuffed tube or excision of a tracheal ring. For this reason, large volume-low pressure and double balloon tubes are advantageous. The double balloon tubes can be inflated and deflated alternately in order to avoid pressure necrosis of the tracheal mucosa. Cuff pressures must be monitored carefully at frequent intervals. It must be remembered that stenoses are not necessarily related directly to inflatable balloons. A recent study by Pearson showed that two-thirds of all tracheal constrictions did appear at the stomal site while one-third did not. Therefore, it is wise to recall that this opening should not be made too large.

Late hemorrhage may follow chronic erosion of the tube into the tracheal mucosa. Therefore, the tube must rest easily within the lumen and should not be too large.

Tracheoesophageal fistulae may occur if the pressure in the cuff is too high causing an ischemic necrosis of the mucosa with subsequent tracheitis. The addition of the nasogastric tube in the esophagus will increase the likelihood since it provides a firm buttress for the tracheostomy tube cuff to squeeze against.

# REMOVING THE TUBE

Despite its lifesaving features, the tracheostomy tube can be a perpetual source of problems as long as it is in place. Removal should be prompt whenever its need has passed. A fenestrated tube can, on occasion, be used as an interim device. If the patient remains comfortable, simply extract the tube and tape the stomal edges shut with a gauze dressing or adhesive tape. Secretions will continue to be coughed through the stoma for 2–3 days, but skin closure takes place in 4–7 days. Occasionally, patients become dependent on tracheostomy tubes, in which case their removal becomes prolonged and difficult. Frequently, it is not possible to remove a tracheostomy from a child until they have grown enough to have a trachea of sufficient diameter to allow more normal airflow characteristics.

### Selected References for Further Reading

1. Borman, J. and Davidson, J. T. A history of tracheostomy. *Brit. J. Anaesth. 35:* 388, 1963.
2. Dugan, D. J. and Samson, P. C. Tracheostomy: present day indications and techniques. *Amer. J. Surg. 106:* 290–295, 1963.

3. Eiseman, B. and Spencer, F. C. Tracheostomy: an underrated surgical procedure. *J.A.M.A. 184:* 684–687, 1963.

4. Grillo, H. C. Surgery of the trachea. *Curr. Probl. Surg.* 3–59, July, 1970.

5. Grillo, H. C., Cooper, J. D., Geffin, B., and Pontoppidan, H. A low-pressure cuff for tracheostomy tubes to minimize tracheal injury: a comparative clinical trial. *J. Thorac. Cardiovasc. Surg. 62:* 898–907, 1971.

6. Jackson, C. High tracheostomy and other errors the chief causes of chronic laryngeal stenosis. *Surg. Gynec. Obstet. 32:* 392, 1921.

7. McClelland, R. M. A. Complications of tracheostomy. *Brit. Med. J. 2:* 567, 1965.

8. Meade, J. W. Tracheostomy: its complications and their management. *New Eng. J. Med. 265:* 519–523, 1961.

9. Mulder, D. S. and Fox, C. L. Complications of tracheostomy: relationship to long-term ventilatory assistance. *Trauma 9:* 389–402, 1969.

10. Pearson, F. G., Goldberg, M., and daSilva, A. J. Tracheal stenosis complicating tracheostomy with cuffed tubes. *Arch. Surg. 97:* 380–394, 1968.

11. Shelly, W. M., Dawson, R. B., and May, I. A. Cuffed tubes as a cause of tracheal stenosis. *J. Thorac. Cardiovasc. Surg. 57:* 623–627, 1969.

12. Toy, F. J. and Weinstein, J. D. A percutaneous tracheostomy device. *Surgery 65:* 384–389, 1979.

# THIRTEEN

# Ventilators

Ventilators are mechanical transport mechanisms for the introduction of gases into the respiratory tract at varying pressures and volumes. The natural process of respiration includes both the transport of gases to and across the alveolar-capillary membrane and the sequence of physiologic mechanisms related to their exchange for tissue utilization. This chapter introduces the basic concepts of ventilator care, but leaves the remainder of respiration physiology to more complete volumes dealing with pulmonary medicine.

## INDICATIONS FOR USING VENTILATORS

A ventilator should be used whenever clinical circumstances or laboratory studies suggest that the patient cannot ventilate adequately by himself. It is very important to anticipate the need for ventilator assistance rather than wait until the need is made obvious by signs of impending respiratory failure. Whenever ventilatory assistance is delayed until there is clear evidence of respiratory failure, lung tissue is often altered irreversibly. It may be possible to predict that a patient will or may do badly if left to breathe on his own from a consideration of the type of operation or anesthesia contemplated. A technique that utilizes large doses of potent respiratory depressants such as morphine, or a major abdominal operation in an obese patient with chronic lung disease present good examples of situations in which the decision to ventilate the patient post-operatively can be made well in advance. Additional clinical indications include cardiac arrest, flail chest, multiple injury (two or more organ systems or three or more organs), peritonitis, prolonged shock, CNS depression (from drugs, infection, or trauma), severe pulmonary disease, massive smoke inhalation, and aspiration of vomitus.

Laboratory values may indicate a need for ventilatory assistance in critically ill or injured patients. Deteriorating arterial blood gases on room air ($pO_2$ < 55 mm Hg; $pCO_2$ > 60 mm Hg) or 40% oxygen ($pO_2$ < 60 mm Hg), physiological shunting within the lung of 40% or more or an alveolar-arterial oxygen difference (>55 mm Hg on room air) all suggest the need for ventilatory assistance.

Pulmonary function tests may also provide indications for ventilatory support (e.g. decreasing tidal volume).

Some relatively simple objective criteria are presented in Table 13.1. Probably as important as the quantitative criteria are the qualitative criteria particularly the establishment of trended data. Initially a patient may well be able to produce "good numbers," but the critical evaluation may be a clinical one, such as whether the patient is likely to become tired in the middle of the night and be unable to continue working as hard.

## EQUIPMENT

Ventilators can be divided into two categories: *pressure-limited* and *volume-limited*. Both kind of devices act directly through the normal or surgical pathways of gas flow (naso-oropharyngeal or tracheal) into the lung using positive pressure mechanisms. The equipment is designed for minimal interference to access to the patient by the physicians and other health professionals. In practice, volume-cycled machines are used in nearly all situations where mechanical ventilation is needed for more than one or two hours. The exception to this rule is in the neonatal ICU where pressure-cycled machines are extensively used.

**Table 13.1  Quantitative Criteria for Intervention**

| | | Acceptable Range | Conservative[a] Therapy Indicated | Intubation and Mechanical Ventilation Indicated |
|---|---|---|---|---|
| Mechanical | Respiratory rate | 15–25 | 25–35 | Over 35 |
| | Vital capacity, ml/kg | 70–30 | 30–15 | Less than 15 |
| | Insp. force cm water | 100–50 | 50–25 | Less than 25 |
| Oxygenation | A-aDO$_2$ on 100% | 50–200 | 200–350 | Over 350 |
| | PaO$_2$ Room air | Over 70 | 70–55 | Less than 55 |
| | 100% | Over 400 | 400–323 | Less than 323 |
| | Respiratory index | 0–2 | 2–4? | >4 |
| Ventilation | VD/VT | 0.3–0.4 | 0.4–0.6 | Over 0.6 |
| | PaCO$_2$ mm Hg | 35–45 | 45–60 | Over 60 |
| Work | Total work/min kg M | Less than 0.85 | 0.85–1.80 | Over 1.80 |
| | Total work/L kg M | Less than 0.08 | 0.08–0.18 | Over 0.18 |
| | Resistive work/min kg M | Less than 0.5 | 0.5–1.0 | Over 1.0 |
| | Compliance ml/cm | 100–75 | 75–50 | Less than 50 |
| | Resistance cm/L/sec | Less than 10 | 10–13 | Over 13 |

[a] Conservative therapy: Oxygen, chest physiotherapy, diuretics, bronchodilators, careful monitoring and possible intubation. (From L. A. Rauscher.)

The critically ill or injured patient who requires ventilatory assistance will usually function better on a volume-limited ventilation (Fig. 13.1). These ventilators deliver a set volume of gas without regard for the pressure required (given that one must set limits on that pressure). Volume-limited ventilators are especially valuable if there is significant respiratory difficulty or increased resistance to air flow. The peak flow rates, however, must be adjusted to levels that will not cause excessive turbulence.

Pressure-limited ventilators (Fig. 13.2) on the other hand find usefulness whenever the patient's pulmonary difficulty is minimal, lung compliance is relatively normal, the chest wall is stable, and mental status is alert and cooperative. Generally, it is much easier for the patient to synchronize with the pressure-limited ventilators, but the quantity of ventilation obtained is limited. In these ventilators, the mechanism is set to deliver a certain pressure of gas without regard for the volume of gas delivered. Thus, for bronchospasm or for partial bronchial obstruction, the tidal volume may fall to dangerous levels before it is detected because of the pressure cut-off system. Some experts feel that the greatest asset of the pressure-limited ventilator is its ability to deliver aerosolized drugs!

A comparison of these two types follows:

| *Pressure Cycled* | *Volume Cycled* |
| --- | --- |
| Compensates for leaks | Does not compensate for leaks |
| Does not compensate for changes in compliance | Compensates for changes in compliance |
| Small, relatively inexpensive | Large, expensive |
| Requires compressed gas supplies ($O_2$ + air) | Usually requires $O_2$ only |
| Poor alarm systems | Poor alarm systems |

The choice of individual volume ventilators is large. There are differences between individual ventilators that are probably only of importance in a few patients, such as the need for variation in flow pattern. However, there are major differences

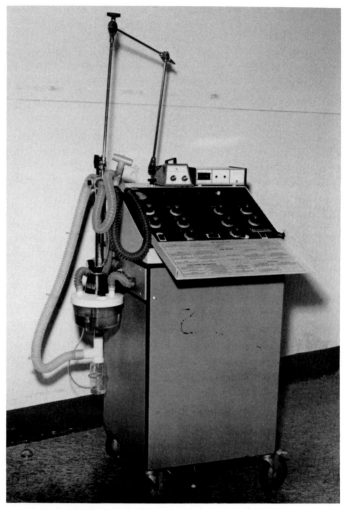

**Figure 13.1.** Volume-limited ventilator.

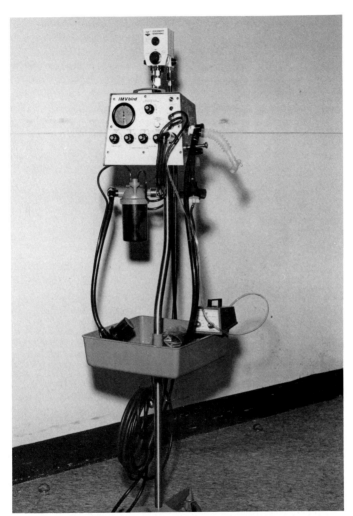

**Figure 13.2.** Pressure-limited ventilator.

in the quality of engineering, maintenance requirements, and efficiency of alarm systems. The brand of ventilator selected for use becomes an administrative decision usually beyond your control, but a decision for pressure- versus volume-limited ventilator is one you can and should become involved in. Meanwhile, try to become an "expert" with the machines available for use in your institution. The ideal, all purpose ventilator probably does not exist at this time.

## MANAGEMENT

Once a ventilator is selected, you will need to determine the pressure and volume ranges to be used, respiratory rate, inspiratory flow rate, concentration of gases to be delivered, how these gases will be humidified and whether any special features (e.g. PEEP, CPAP, sighing) will be needed.

The pressure required to inflate the lungs properly varies greatly from patient to patient and is largely dependent on the tidal volume to be used, the cooperation of the patient, and the resistance of the airway, lungs, and chest wall. Inflation pressures below 30 cm $H_2O$ are relatively safe, whereas inflation pressures greater than 45 cm $H_2O$ lead to an increased risk of alveolar rupture with a resultant pneumothorax. However, in patients with severe bronchospasm, interstitial fibrosis, or congestive atelectasis, higher pressures may be required.

The patients with severe trauma, sepsis, or shock should have a tidal volume of at least 12 to 15 ml/kg body weight. If a pressure of >60 cm $H_2O$ is required to achieve this amount of inflation, one must decide if he is willing to accept a higher risk of pneumothorax or whether the patient can get by on a lower tidal volume (with adequate blood gases). Sometimes the use of PEEP in noncompliant patients will reduce peak airway pressures. The only situation where tidal volumes differ is in the patient with emphysema and a high functional reserve capacity (FRC) where weaning the patient from mechanical ventilation may be much more difficult following 12–15 ml/kg, and volumes of 7–10 ml/kg are used.

A respiratory rate of 8 to 12 per minute is ideal in most patients, particularly if high tidal volumes are used. Many seriously ill patients will be severely tachypneic regardless of the minute ventilation or blood gases and require medication (e.g. morphine, Diazepam) and muscle relaxants (e.g. Panumonium) to synchronize properly with the ventilator. With fixed tidal volume ventilation, changes in $PaCO_2$ are effected by changing rate and therefore minute ventilation. In the course of a patient's illness, other factors which may change $PaCO_2$ are changes in dead space ventilation and $CO_2$ production, and an appropriate response to changing $PaCO_2$ tensions is to change only the rate. The rate control can therefore simplistically be called the $PaCO_2$ control.

An important development in the technique of mechanical ventilation has been the employment of intermittent mandatory ventilation (IMV). This system allows the patient to breathe with a minimum of effort between so-called mandatory mechanical ventilations; the gas inspired during such spontaneous activity has the same $F_IO_2$ as the ventilator gas without rebreathing of expired gas. The "dose" of mechanical ventilation can thus be adjusted commensurate with the patient's ability to do some of the work. The technical requirements of an IMV system demand that:

(a) The ventilator can cycle at very low rates (to one breath in two minutes).

(b) The ventilator circuit can deliver fresh gas at a flow rate and volume equal to that of the patient's need during spontaneous respiration. This is usually achieved by either a very sensitive demand valve within the circuit, or a low-resistance one-way valve within the circuit connected to a fresh gas source.

Inspiratory flow rate control on a volume ventilator allows inspiratory time to be changed. A slow inspiratory flow rate increases inspiratory time and therefore decreases expiratory time and hence venous return. A high inspiratory flow rate may increase inspiratory pressures and increase the incidence of pulmonary barotrauma. The compromise setting seems to be about 50 liters/min or an inspiratory time of one second.

Patients with small airway disease may require longer inspiratory times or lower flow rates to avoid turbulence in narrow small airways.

The gases most frequently used in ventilation are oxygen and compressed air. In most situations, the injured patient needs ventilatory assistance, and additional oxygen is usually only a secondary consideration. Wherever possible, the oxygen concentration is limited to the minimum required to provide reasonable oxygenation of the blood. High concentrations of oxygen ($>50\%$) can be damaging to the lungs depending on the period of exposure. Oxygen toxicity is a very real concern in many patients who are critically ill for long periods of time. Attempt to keep the arterial $pO_2$ in the range of 70 to 100 mm Hg, using as little oxygen in the inhaled gas mixtures as possible. Examination of the relationship between $PaO_2$ and $F_IO_2$ in patients with a range of intrapulmonary shunt fractions shows that where shunts exceed about $40\%$, there is little increase in $PaO_2$ with increasing $F_IO_2$. If hypoxemia is all due to intrapulmonary shunt, there is little need for inspired oxygen concentrations above $50\%$. A more rational approach to this form of hypoxemia, which is by far the commonest finding in hypoxemic patients without intracardiac shunts, is to change the patient from a high to a lower shunt fraction. In the main, this is achieved by the manipulation of FRC and its relationship to closing volume. Ideally, FRC should consistently be higher than closing volume.

Therefore, a rational approach to hypoxemia is:

(a) Exclude hypoxemia due to very low mixed venous oxygen tensions secondary to low or relatively low cardiac output.

(b) Increase FRC by titrating PEEP (positive end expiratory pressure during mechanical ventilation) or CPAP (positive end-expiratory and inspiratory pressure during spontaneous respiration).

(c) Maintain $F_IO_2$ below $50\%$ at all times.

The principal harmful physiologic effect of PEEP/CPAP is reduction of cardiac output, reflecting a relative hypovolemia. Such effects can be managed by volume loading. Evaluation of oxygenation status other than simply maintaining physiologic $PaO_2$ is essential in managing oxygen therapy and PEEP/ CPAP levels. Ideally, the actual shunt should be measured, but since this requires invasive pulmonary artery catheterization, the respiratory index $\left(\dfrac{PAO_2 - PaO_2}{PaO_2}\right)$ which has a close correlation with shunt fraction, but requires only a knowledge of the $F_IO_2$, the $PaCO_2$, and the $PaO_2$ and an estimate of the barometric pressure can be used. The equation is:

$$R.I. = \frac{P(AaDO_2)}{PaO_2}$$
$$= \frac{[F_IO_2 \text{ (Barometric pressure} - SVP_{H_2O}^{37°})\text{-}PaCO_2]\text{-}PaO_2}{PaO_2}$$

A clinically accurate calculation of the shunt is $Qs/Qt = 5.8(RI) + 6.7$.

As far as pathophysiology is concerned, the lower the respiratory index (RI) the better. The index allows multiple changes to be made at the same time with an objective assessment of the effects of such maneuvers.

Positive end expiratory pressure (PEEP) has been used to improve oxygenation and prevent or treat the atelectasis which almost inevitably develops in many critically ill and injured patients. Many ventilators have adjustable PEEP built into the machine or CPAP can be provided by attaching tubing to the expiratory port and then placing the other end of the tubing under 5 to 10 cm of water. The pressures can be varied according to the need, but pressures exceeding 10 cm $H_2O$ are not tolerated very well by the patient. The best results are obtained when the PEEP level is titrated against intrapulmonary shunt and cardiac output (approximately 5 to 8 cm $H_2O$). Patients generally tolerate increasing PEEP if only 1 to 2 cm $H_2O$ pressure are added at a time and should be weaned at similar increments. When the pressures exceed 15 cm $H_2O$, great care must be taken to provide adequate circulatory volume support or the patient may enter profound shock because of relative hypovolemia and decreased venous return to the right side of the heart. Moreover, all health professionals caring for patients on ventilators with high PEEP should be prepared to diagnose and treat pneumothorax (some even feel prophylactic chest tubes are in order!).

Give the maximum humidity possible because of the extraordinary drying effect that most ventilators have on the tracheobronchial tree. In small patients, however, particularly those with heart disease or inhalation injuries, some of the newer machines can provide so much moisture that the quantity of fluid absorbed through the alveoli and bronchial mucosa may actually overload the circulation and cause congestive heart failure. If the gases are warmed by the machine to temperatures approaching humidity and less, moisture will be needed. Careful observation of the thickness or dryness of the bronchial secretions, correlated with the patient's weight and vital signs, should allow physicians to determine the ideal amount of humidification.

Most volume-limited machines have a sighing mechanism. Under normal circumstances, all people unconsciously and involuntarily take several deep breaths each hour. This hyperinflation of the lungs, referred to as sighing, inflates many of the alveoli that are not expanded by ordinary tidal volumes. When a patient is placed on a ventilator, especially of the volume-limited type, the resultant fixed tidal volume, if provided at low volume for prolonged periods, will allow atelectasis to develop in those areas that are poorly ventilated. To prevent this from occurring, it is important to hyperinflate the lungs for two to three breaths with a tidal volume that is 1½ to 2 times greater, providing, of course, that the inflation pressures do not exceed 50 to 60 cm $H_2O$. The optimum frequency of sighing varies from patient to patient, but 6 to 12 times per hour appears to be satisfactory for most patients. Now that larger tidal volumes are used (12–15 ml/kg) the sigh does not affect the development of atelectasis or a progressive reduction of FRC occurring in critically ill patients. In effect, the patient gets a sigh with every breath and the use of "additional" sighs under these conditions produces very high airway pressures with the consequent increased risk of pulmonary barotrauma.

# COMPLICATIONS

There are some distinct disadvantages of the in-line machines. Of primary importance is the hazard of bacterial contamination of the respiratory tract from the equipment or because of interference with the cough reflex and the activity of the mucocillary blanket and alveolar macrophages. Therefore, sterilization of nebulizers and ventilators is of great importance. The basis for all sterilization lies in vigorous mechanical cleansing including scrubbing with a brush and rinsing with copious amounts of water as soon after use as possible. The use of ethylene oxide sterilization may not be adequate. Various chemical soaks have been recommended. The best solution is the use of disposable tubing and other parts that may be exposed to bacterial and viral contamination. Unfortunately, the cost factor for these disposable items is high.

When the patient is first placed on a ventilator, there may be difficulty synchronizing the machine with his efforts to breathe, especially when a volume respirator is used. A first step is to attempt to remove the patient's drive or stimulus to breathe. This may include lowering the $pCO_2$ to less than 25 to 30 mm Hg and raising the $PO_2$ to over 100 mm Hg. IMV has reduced the need for complete control of respiration. In some cases, large doses of sedatives such as morphine, Diazepam, chlorpromazine, and $MgSO4$ may be required. If these maneuvers and drugs are not successful, muscle paralyzers such as succinylcholine or curare may be required (e.g. deliberate hyperventilation for intracranial hypertension where intracranial compliance is low, in tetanus, etc.). In general, it is easier for patients to synchronize with the pressure-limited ventilators, but these respirators may not provide adequate ventilation if partial obstruction develops. Furthermore, increased intrapulmonary pressures may cause rupture of alveoli resulting in a pneumothorax with or without mediastinal and cervical emphysema and increased intrathoracic pressure leading to a decreased venous return to the right side of the heart.

When large tidal volumes are used, particularly if the patient's respiratory rate is high, the resultant high minute ventilation may cause a severe respiratory alkalosis. In addition to the acid-base problems that may result, an arterial $pCO_2$ below 20 to 25 mm Hg may cause severe vasoconstriction in cerebral vessels. On the other hand, if the $pCO_2$ is allowed to rise above 40 to 45 mm Hg, the hypercarbia may stimulate the patient's respiratory center causing him to take extra breaths out of phase with the ventilator. As a consequence, one should attempt to maintain an arterial $pCO_2$ of 30 to 35 mm Hg.

In many patients, particularly those with sepsis, it will be extremely difficult to keep the arterial $pCO_2$ above 30 mm Hg. The three possible methods currently available for correcting such hypocarbia include reducing the tidal volume, reducing the respiratory rate, or adding dead space between the ventilator and the patient. Since a high tidal volume is preferred and since many patients will remain tachypneic in spite of large doses of Diazepam, morphine, and $MgSO_4$, one may have to add dead space to a patient circuit on many machines (newer machines with a continuous variable rate may not require dead space). The dead space is added in increments of 50 ml and is adjusted according to the arterial $P_{CO_2}$, allowing at least 15 minutes for the blood gases to stabilize after each increment is added. Although 100 to 200 ml of dead space is used frequently, more than 300 ml is seldom tolerated by the patient, perhaps because of the additional pressure required to expel the gas from the lung through the increased length of tubing. Fortunately, such machines are being superceded by machines with a continuously variable rate, and with IMV rates down to one in three minutes so that addition of dead space becomes unnecessary. Furthermore, since one of the commonest hazards facing the patient on a mechanical ventilator is accidental disconnection, the addition of further complexity to the circuit is counter-productive particularly since most circuits are held together only by friction.

Simple bedside evaluation of the patient's ventilatory status by serial vital capacity, inspiratory force, respiratory rate, respiratory index and $PaCO_2$ measurements will determine when the patient can be weaned from the ventilator. Weaning is a problem that has been made somewhat easier (almost automatic) by the addition of IMV. The IMV rate is slowly decreased while allowing the patient to begin to ventilate on his own. Many machines synchronize the patient's own respiratory rate with that of the machine and the IMV rate is reduced gradually until the patient ventilates entirely on his own with insignificant changes in pulmonary parameters. Attention must be paid however to the presence of:

(a) Systemic disease which has not responded to therapy (heart failure, etc.)

(b) Signs of exhaustion from the increased work of breathing or from sleep deficiency.

(c) A catabolic state resulting from inadequate nutrition during the illness

Weaning from mechanical ventilation should be regarded as a separate process from weaning from therapy designed to maintain oxygenation. Many patients are able to tolerate a large reduction in ventilator rate, but remain in need of high PEEP/CPAP levels. Many patients can be successfully weaned from both the ventilator and PEEP/CPAP but still are unable to protect their airway and must therefore remain intubated. These three processes should be managed independently.

It is probably better to wean the inspired oxygen concentration down from 50% to 30% in stages before reducing PEEP/CPAP levels, unless these levels are very high. Once the patient is stable on 30% oxygen, then the PEEP/CPAP level can be progressively reduced to 5 cm water.

Ideally, patients being weaned should continue to have a few centimeters of CPAP (5 cm water) until extubated. This maneuver is associated with an improvement in oxygenation and maintenance of FRC at a crucial period of their illness. This low level of CPAP has not been associated with any serious hazard.

The duration of the weaning process is highly variable. It may be convenient to have the patient weaned before a weekend, but some patients do very badly if weaned more rapidly than a reduction of IMV rate of one per day. This is particularly true at the lower end of the IMV scale where a reduction of IMV rate from 2/min to 1/min represents a reduction of 50% in mechanical contribution.

With careful attention to detail, ventilators have become an invaluable asset in the management of the critical ill or injured patient.

### Selected References for Further Reading

1. Ashbaugh, D. G., Bigelow, D. B., Petty, T. L. and Levine, B. E. Acute respiratory distress in adults. *Lancet 2:* 319, 1967.

2. Benumof, J. L., Raushcer, A. and Herren, A. Comparison of respiratory index [P(AaDO$_2$)/PaO$_2$] with transpulmonary shunt. Proceedings American Society of Anesthesiology, pp. 185–186, 1977.

3. Campbell, G. S. Respiratory failure in surgical patients. Current Problems in Surgery, February, 1976.

4. Downs, J. B., Klein, E. F., Jr., Desautels, D., Modell, J. H. and Kirby, R. R. Intermittent mandatory ventilation: a new approach to weaning patients from mechanical ventilation. *Chest 64:* 331, 1973.

5. Gregory, G. A., Kitterman, J. A., Phibbs, R. H., Tooley, W. H. and Hamilton, W. K. Treatment of the idiopathic respiratory distress syndrome with continuous positive airway pressure. *New Engl. J. Med. 284:* 1333, 1971.

6. Harken, A. H., Brennan, M. F., Smith, B. and Barsamian, E. M. The hemodynamic response to positive end-expiratory ventilation in hypovolemic patients. *Surgery 76:* 786, 1974.

7. Kirby, R. P., Downs, J. B., Civeta, J. M., Modell, J. H., Dannemiller, F. J., Klein, E. F. and Hodges, M. High level positive end-expiratory pressure (PEEP) in acute respiratory insufficiency. *Chest 67:* 156, 1975.

8. Klein, E. F., Jr. Weaning from mechanical breathing with intermittent mandatory ventilation. *Arch. Surg. 110:* 345, 1975.

9. Laver, M. B., Morgan, J. Bendixen, H. H. and Radford, E. P., Jr. Lung volume, compliance and arterial oxygen tensions during controlled ventilation. *J. Appl. Physiol. 19:* 725, 1964.

10. McConnell, D. H., Maloney, J. V., Jr. and Buckberg, G. D. Post-operative intermittent positive pressure breathing treatments; physiological considerations. *J. Thorac. Cardiovasc. Surg. 68:* 944, 1974.

11. Petty, T. L., Acute respiratory failure in surgical patients. *Contemp. Surg. 5:* 9–11, 1974.

12. Powers, S. R. The use of positive end-expiratory pressure (PEEP) for respiratory support. *Surg. Clin. N. Amer. 54:* 1125, 1974.

13. Sahn, S. A., Lakshminarayan, S. and Petty, T. L. Weaning from mechanical ventilation. *J.A.M.A. 235:* 2208–2212, 1976.

14. Spencer, F. C., Benson, D. W. and Lin, W. C. Use of mechanical respiratory in the management of respiratory insufficiency following trauma or operation for cardiac or pulmonary disease. *J. Thorac. Cardiovasc. Surg. 38:* 758, 1959.

15. Suster, P. M., Fairley, H. B. and Isenberg, M. D. Optimum end-expiratory pressure in patients with acute pulmonary failure. *New Engl. J. Med. 292:* 284–289, 1975.

16. Zwillich, C. W., Pierson, D. J., Creagh, E., Sutton, F. D., Schatz, E. and Petty, T. L. Complications of assisted ventilation, a prospective study of 354 consecutive episodes. *Amer. J. Med. 57:* 161–170, 1974.

# FOURTEEN

# Gastrointestinal Intubation

The ability to pass a flexible rubber or plastic tube into the stomach permits the physician to achieve a wide variety of diagnostic and therapeutic goals. Without gastric decompression, the surgeon's ability to safely perform many abdominal operations would be severely hindered, and without access to the secretory products of the gastrointestinal tract, the gastroenterologist's diagnostic capability would not be nearly as efficient. Gastrointestinal intubation is therefore one of the most useful and frequently performed of all clinical procedures. This chapter discusses not only the basic technique of gastric intubation but also describes specific applications such as gastric analysis, gastric lavage, gastric feeding, intestinal decompression, and balloon tamponage of bleeding esophageal varices.

## HISTORY

Perhaps the earliest recorded attempt to pass something into the human stomach occurred during Roman times when it was fashionable among the aristocracy to induce emesis in order to be able to extend their feasts throughout the day. For this purpose, a strip of leather, known as a "lorum vomitorum" was coated with noxious substances and swallowed. Shortly thereafter, the tube and gastric contents were expelled, and presumably the next course was then served. In the 16th century, Ambroise Pare passed the stalk of a leek into the stomach, but his purpose was never clearly revealed. Herman Boerhaave suggested that a flexible tube might be passed into the stomach in his writings but there is no record of the deed. John Hunter thought that "balsams and oils" might be conveyed into the stomach of drowned persons in order to revive them. Whether his plan ever achieved success is doubtful, but he did report a man with paralyzed muscles of deglutition who was maintained with tube feedings.

In America, Phillip Syng Physik introduced the gastric tube and pump around 1800. Although not the first to intubate the stomach, he was the first to perform gastric lavage for cases of poison ingestion. During the remainder of the 19th century, only minor improvements were made; Ewald's introduction of soft rubber is perhaps most notable.

At the beginning of the 20th century, when tubes could easily be passed into the stomach, attention turned to the duodenum. During 1909, Einhorn reported a simple method of reaching the duodenum by using a tube with a weighted tip. Many variations of this principle were introduced but, in 1921, Levin introduced a small soft rubber catheter with a rounded but unweighted tip which he found would pass through the pylorus just as easily as weighted varieties. The Levin tube was quickly accepted and retains its popularity today. Vented tubes (e.g. Salem sumps) are effective and permit aspiration without blockage by stomach contents.

## EQUIPMENT

The type of tube selected naturally depends on the purpose for which it is intended. Salem tubes incorporating the sump principle are commonly used for gastric decompression. Fine soft plastic tubes are well tolerated for gastric feeding. The larger Ewald tubes are better suited for gastric irrigation, particularly in the event of acute upper gastrointestinal hemorrhage when large volumes of iced saline must be introduced and blood clots must be aspirated.

Adults require No. 14–18 Fr tubes, whereas Nos. 10–12 Fr

are appropriate for infants. Rubber tubes are softer and more comfortable but are more difficult to pass since they lack rigidity and tend to coil within the hypopharynx. Plastic tubes, on the other hand, are firmer and easier to pass (since they become exceptionally rigid with chilling). Some plastic tubes have the added advantage of incorporating radiopaque markings and may thus be localized by x-ray.

The number of suction holes deserves special attention. Some tubes have as many as nine and are therefore ideal for gastric drainage. Be careful, however, not to pass one of these into a child, since the proximal hole may lie in the lower pharynx and prevent effective suction. Other tubes have as few as four holes and are much less efficient. Extra holes may be cut but they should not be too large or the wall will be weakened. Sump tubes (those with an auxiliary channel) are less likely to obstruct.

In addition to the appropriate tube, other necessary items include a syringe (large plunger type is preferable to bulb syringe since stronger suction may be applied), a small basin, aqueous lubricant, adhesive tape, a clamp, and saline for irrigation.

---

## NEEDED FOR GASTRIC INTUBATION:

| | |
|---|---|
| Nasogastric tube (Levin, Salem, etc.) | Saline for irrigation |
| | Small basin |
| Glass of water and straw | Adhesive tape |
| Aqueous lubricant | Clamp |
| 50-cc syringe | Suction apparatus |

---

## TECHNIQUE

Assume that this is the patient's first experience with gastric intubation and begin with a careful explanation of the need for the procedure. Avoid the vernacular (e.g. "I'm going to pass a red snake") because careless terminology not only insults the patient's intelligence, but also produces fear and anxiety. The purpose and importance of the tube should be heavily stressed because the patient will then be less likely to remove the tube prematurely.

Nasogastric tubes, as their name implies, are usually passed transnasally. The patient, however, does not realize this and may not even be aware that the nose and throat communicate. These facts must therefore be explained, emphasizing that there will be less drooling, gagging, and vomiting. Furthermore, speech will not be altered and there will be no opportunity to bite or chew the tube.

Occasionally patients have obstruction of the nares to a degree that prohibits the passage of a tube. In such cases, the mouth may be used, but a plastic airway must be kept between the teeth when the patient is asleep or unconscious so that the lumen will remain patent.

Ask the patient to sit up or else raise the head of his bed approximately 30°. Pour a glass of water and ask him to take a mouthful, hold it in the pharynx, and swallow only after directed to do so. Most patients swallow too soon so a trial run is useful. Coat the tip of the tube with an aqueous lubricant and pass it through the nostril and into the nasopharynx. Elevating the tip of the nose aids in this process.

There are two potential sites of obstruction at this point. First, septal deviation may severely limit the nostril, in which case the opposite side should be used. If both are tight, Neo-Synephrine or ephedrine spray may help. Pain may be alleviated by using 1% topical Pontocaine or 4% Lidocaine. Second, the posterior wall of the nasopharynx may present a firm barrier to the tip of the tube. Turn or extend the head in order to pass this point. If difficulty persists, use an iced plastic tube and mold the tip into a gentle curve before introduction.

As the tube enters the pharynx, stimulation of vagal nerve fibers results in a reflex cough. Pause, reassure the patient, and ask him to breathe deeply. Ask him to take a mouthful of water and hold it as he practiced. Advance the tube 5–10 cm as you ask the patient to swallow and the tip should pass directly into the esophagus. With a second mouthful, advance another 5–10 cm and continue until the stomach is reached. An alternate method is to use a straw and have the patient drink continuously as the tube is passed.

Vigorous coughing, a change of complexion, or a change of voice usually indicates tracheal intubation in which case the tip should be withdrawn to the pharynx. Try again after the patient quiets down. Do not allow the patient to reach up and remove the tube completely!

There are many ways to determine when the tube reaches the stomach. First, the tube has marks, usually three, signifying when the tip has reached the esophagogastric junction, antrum, and pylorus, but this is not the best guide since patients vary in size and tubes may coil within the esophagus. Air, 10 cc, may be injected into the tube while a stethoscope is placed over the left upper quadrant to detect the resultant sounds. However, the most useful method by far is the aspiration of gastric juice. Moreover, if most of a volume of swallowed fluid can be removed, then you can be reasonably confident that the tip lies in a suitable location for drainage.

## TUBE MAINTENANCE

Once assured that the tube is well positioned, as proven by the ability to aspirate most of a swallowed volume of water, it should be fixed to the nose with adhesive tape. Care must be taken to allow sufficient slack to prevent pressure necrosis of the alar skin and cartilage.

Careful nursing orders must be written to assure continued tube function. Unlike the chest cavity which requires constant suction, the gastrointestinal tract should be drained with a cycled or intermittent suction apparatus. Modern suction machines usually have two settings, −9 and −12 cm of $H_2O$. This means that the machine shuts off for a brief period of time whenever the selected level is reached. If there is fluid to be drained, negative pressure remains below the preset limit. Once drainage has occurred, mucosa is drawn against the tube surface, the pressure rises, and suction is temporarily interrupted. Assuming that the suction pump is functioning efficiently, the lower setting is adequate for gastric suction. For the vented tubes (Salem sump) constant suction works equally well.

Nasogastric tubes must be irrigated with small volumes of saline at least every 4 hours and any other time that they appear to be occluded or functioning poorly. Keep a syringe and saline by the bedside and adopt the habit of checking the tube's position and function each time that the patient is seen. If there is poor return of instilled saline, adjust the position of the tube in order to avoid being called by the nurse later because of malfunction. Another check is to have the patient drink some water (saline tastes bad) and see if it is aspirated. Patients like this, too, because it moistens the throat. All gastrointestinal fluid aspirated should be measured as well as saved until it is observed by a physician. If patients are disoriented or oversedated, they may prematurely remove the tube unless their hands are restrained. Close attention to respiratory function is also important since anyone with a tube in his pharynx is more susceptible to pulmonary complications.

## SPECIAL PROBLEMS

### Gastric Feeding

Nasogastric tubes are sometimes necessary for feeding debilitated patients. Use either a standard Levin tube or Salem sump or a shorter feeding tube which extends to the lower esophagus. The shorter tube, by failing to pass through the cardioesophageal junction, does not cause acid reflux or symptoms of esophagitis nearly to the extent that the Levin tube will. However, there is one disadvantage; namely, correct positioning cannot be confirmed by the aspiration of gastric juice. Unconscious patients present a special problem in this regard since there must be absolute certainty of the correct placement of the tube in order to avoid instillation of food into their tracheas. Remember that comatose patients may have no cough reflex to indicate misplacement of the tube.

Small, soft, polyethylene feeding tubes are now available which produce minimal discomfort but are exceedingly difficult to insert. One way to facilitate placement is to insert the tips of a feeding catheter and a No. 16 Fr Levin tube into one-half of an empty gelatin capsule (the red half of a 65-mg Darvon compound capsule is the ideal size) (Fig. 14.1). Pass both tubes into the stomach together, wait a few minutes for the gelatin capsule to dissolve, and then slowly withdraw the Levin tube. The feeding catheter should remain in the stomach and may be left there for several days with very little discomfort being experienced by the patient. Many varieties of weighted feeding tubes are now available.

Two complications which are specifically associated with gastric feeding are aspiration and diarrhea. The first may be prevented by inserting the tube properly, and feeding the patient slowly during waking hours with his head elevated. Rapid infusion at night with the patient supine and asleep merely increases the risk of aspiration. The tube feedings can be accomplished in two ways. The first is by constant flow using a constant flow pump (e.g. IVAC, Holter, etc.) 24 hours/day. The second is by hourly feedings of a set amount, checking the residual in the stomach before each feeding. Diarrhea is related not only to the volume and speed of infusion but also to the composition of the feeding solution. If diarrhea continues after the infusion rate is decreased, a change in feeding formula

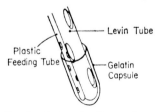

**Figure 14.1.** Small polyethylene feeding catheters can be introduced more easily if passed along with a Levin tube.

may be necessary. Bulk laxatives (e.g. Metamucil) may be used to ameliorate this problem.

## Gastric Analysis

The analysis of gastric fluid may serve many useful purposes including determination of absent or excessive acidity, measurement of residual gastric content, and collection of culture material for the diagnosis of tuberculosis. Gastric juice specimens are best collected in the early morning before the patient has eaten. Samples for AFB culture should be obtained even before the patient brushes his teeth or thinks about breakfast since active peristalsis will promote passage of swallowed sputum into the small intestine.

The presence of acid may be determined by testing a sample of gastric juice with Topfer's reagent or pH paper. If no acid is found, a stimulant such as histamine phosphate (1 mg) should be given in order to determine whether the patient is achlorhydric. Histalog (50 mg) is considered by many to be much safer than histamine because it produces fewer side effects. Quantitative acid determinations are best made on 15-minute aliquots collected over 2- or 12-hour intervals and measured for acidity.

Whenever the gastric aspirate is dark brown or black, always test with guaiac or benzidine for hematin, the presence of which indicates gastrointestinal bleeding.

Patients who are suspected of having pyloric obstruction should have measurements of residual gastric contents in the early morning. The presence of undigested food from the previous day or volumes consistently in excess of 100 cc are indicative of obstruction.

## Gastric Lavage

Gastric lavage may be lifesaving following the accidental ingestion of poisons or drug overdose. A large catheter should be passed promptly and irrigation carried out with 2–3 liters of tap water or saline.

Small volumes (100–200 ml) should be repeatedly injected and removed. Larger volumes will overload the stomach, increase the danger of aspiration, and promote relaxation of the pylorus with resultant passage of the ingested poison into the small intestine.

Certain contraindications to lavage should be remembered. Ingestion of strong acids or caustic alkalis predisposes to perforation after intubation. Lavage is also hazardous when performed on the unconscious patient because of the danger of aspiration. Lavage in these instances should be preceded by endotracheal intubation with inflation of the tracheal balloon in order to isolate the airway from any gastric reflux.

### Gastric Hemorrhage

Patients who are bleeding from the upper gastrointestinal tract require gastric intubation for drainage purposes as well as for monitoring the rate of hemorrhage. There is no rationale for avoiding gastric intubation in bleeding patients because of the fear that the tube might induce additional bleeding sites! The result of gastric hemorrhage without drainage is a stomach distended with blood, hematemesis, a panic-stricken patient, aspiration, and little or no indication of the degree of hemorrhage aside from what may be learned from the vital signs!

When bleeding is active enough to necessitate irrigation with ice water, use a large rubber tube (e.g. Ewald tube). Levin tubes are inadequate because they become easily plugged with clot. Successful irrigation requires two 50-cc syringes and two persons (one injecting and aspirating, another emptying and filling) in order to achieve sufficient hypothermia to decrease the rate of hemorrhage.

If the presumptive diagnosis is hemorrhage from ruptured esophageal varices, or if the cause is not known, and esophagogastroscopy is not immediately available, then balloon tamponade with a Sengstaken-Blakemore or similar tube should be carried out. This is a three-lumen tube, one of which drains the stomach, and the other two lead to esophageal and gastric balloons (Fig. 14.2). In a four-lumen tube, there is an additional aspirating port above the esophageal balloon. Patients who are

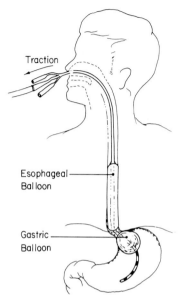

**Figure 14.2.** Sengstaken-Blakemore tube for compression of esophageal varices.

to have a Sengstaken-Blakemore tube inserted, like all gastrointestinal bleeders, should be very well sedated. Vigorously irrigate and empty the stomach beforehand in order to minimize the chance of hematemesis and aspiration during intubation. Lubricate the tube liberally and pass it either transnasally or transorally into the stomach. Inflate the gastric balloon first with 200 ml of air and apply 3 lb of traction to the tube. This is frequently sufficient to stop the bleeding. Continue to irrigate the center lumen and, if the aspirate clears, continue tamponage for 24–48 hours. A Levin tube should be placed into the esophagus alongside the Sengstaken-Blakemore tube to drain swallowed saliva if the four-lumen tube is not used. However, if the bleeding continues, inflate the esophageal balloon with 100–150 ml of air. If hemorrhage still persists, then this is indicative of a lower site of hemorrhage.

## Intestinal Obstruction

In the event of abdominal distention secondary to either mechanical or functional obstruction, a long intestinal tube is often useful. A number of tubes have been designed with features permitting safe and facile passage through the pylorus and into the distended small intestine. Two in particular have remained popular and are discussed here (Fig. 14.3). The Miller-Abbott tube has a double lumen incorporating an inflatable balloon at its tip to permit rapid advancement by peristaltic action. The Cantor tube is a single lumen tube with a large internal diameter (18 Fr) permitting more efficient suction. It relies on a balloon which may be partially filled with mercury to provide weight and encourage intestinal advancement.

Both tubes are passed into the stomach in much the same way as a Levin tube with certain notable modifications. First, it is wise to sedate the patient and prepare the nose with topical Pontocaine in order to ease the discomfort produced by the balloons.

Miller-Abbott tubes will usually pass the nose easily if the balloon is completely deflated and well lubricated. After the tip is in the stomach, inject 5 ml of mercury to encourage the balloon to traverse the pylorus and enter the second portion of the duodenum. When using a Cantor tube, mercury (5 ml) must be injected into the balloon before insertion. Let the

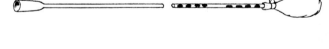

To Balloon

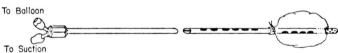

To Suction

**Figure 14.3.** Long intestinal tubes. Above, Cantor tube with single lumen—mercury must be injected into balloon before insertion. Below, Miller-Abbott tube with double lumen—both air and mercury may be injected after insertion.

mercury fall into the balloon neck, fold the balloon tip back over the tube, and then fold it into a cone. Apply lubricant liberally and pass the tube through the nostril. As the balloon reaches the pharynx, the mercury will fall by gravity to a point where it can be swallowed with ease and propelled into the esophagus.

The art of placing long intestinal tubes lies in coaxing the tube through the pylorus. Since the underlying principle is gravity plus a little peristalsis, the patient should be lying on his right side for 2–3 hours. The use of fluoroscopy is of great benefit at this point and should be employed frequently to ensure rapid passage of the tube. The radiologist cannot guarantee cannulation of the pyloric channel, but he can often maneuver the tip into the distal antrum from which point gravity will do the rest. If the balloon is left high in the fundus, it might remain motionless indefinitely. If fluoroscopy cannot be used, frequent abdominal x-rays are necessary to check the position and advancement of the tube.

Once the long intestinal tube enters the duodenum, advance it 15–20 cm every 2 hours until sufficiently introduced into the small intestine. Tape the tube to the nose after each advancement to prevent it from coming back out. If follow-up x-rays show that the tube is coiled within the stomach, then it has been advanced too rapidly and should be partially withdrawn.

Long intestinal tubes must be irrigated periodically to assure lumen patency, but use small volumes and don't always expect to retrieve the injected fluid. Contrary to popular belief, long intestinal tubes may be connected to intermittent suction throughout the period of insertion without hindering peristaltic advancement. Once the tube resides within the small intestine, a Levin tube should be used for gastric decompression. Finally, when removing a long tube, withdraw only 30–45 cm at a time every 30–60 minutes. Never remove the tube in one stage or there may be risk of intussusception or intestinal injury. If firm resistance to extraction is encountered, tape the tube to the nose, come back later, and try again. Very rarely, a long tube cannot be extracted from above and must be cut off at the nares and allowed to pass per rectum.

# COMPLICATIONS

The list of potential complications of gastrointestinal tubes almost exceeds the list of indications for their use, which says something about the great care with which the rather fragile gastrointestinal tract must be intubated. Epistaxis following traumatic transit of the nostrils may be severe enough to require nasal packs. Inappropriate force at a lower level may result in pharyngeal or esophageal perforation, particularly in patients with pathological lesions such as stricture, diverticulum, or neoplasm.

Inaccurate placement of a tube may lead to intratracheal instillation of material intended for the stomach, e.g. tube feeding formula, resulting in severe aspiration pneumonitis. Even minute volumes of oily material (e.g. mineral oil) on the tip of a tube may produce lipoid pneumonia if the trachea is entered. Therefore, only aqueous lubricants should be used.

Patients often vomit during intubation, particularly those experiencing gastrointestinal hemorrhage. Therefore, somnolent or unconscious patients should have their heads lowered in advance to prevent aspiration. Syncope and brachycardia may also be induced by intubation, apparently following stimulation of a vasovagal reflex.

Fluid loss is a predictable consequence of any tube inserted for drainage but it becomes a complication only when these losses are not met with appropriate replacement. Therefore, all fluids drained must be measured accurately and recorded in a systematic manner. It is occasionally helpful to send samples for electrolyte determination to aid replacement calculations. Also, constant ingestion or irrigation of the intubated stomach with large volumes of water may result in significant electrolyte losses.

Considerable discomfort, such as dryness of the mouth, sore throat, and sinusitis, may attend prolonged use of indwelling tubes. In addition, they may occlude or irritate the eustachian tube orifice and produce otitis media. Laryngeal edema and even stenosis have been reported following pressure necrosis and ulceration of the respiratory mucosa. Similar ulcerative lesions may occur in the esophagus and stomach.

Long intestinal tubes produce their own complications, many of which are a result of human error. For example, overdistention of a Miller-Abbott tube balloon (or inadvertent irrigation of the "balloon lumen" rather than the suction lumen) may produce painful distention of a segment of intestine, or even interference with blood supply, necrosis, and finally perforation. Mercury-filled balloons of Cantor tubes have also become overdistended, apparently due to permeation of the balloon by intestinal gases. This latter complication may be avoided by injecting the mercury with a 20- or 21-gauge needle which leaves a hole of sufficient size to allow egress of air but not large enough to permit mercury escape.

Inadequate tube maintenance may result in occlusion of the lumen, either temporarily when particulate matter lodges at the suction orifices or permanently when the tube becomes knotted. Regular irrigation will prevent the first cause. Knotting is a rare but serious complication since it may re-establish the intestinal obstruction for which the long tube was originally inserted. Its occurrence may be prevented by avoiding the excessive tube slack in the gastric fundus. Remember to deflate the air-filled balloons before removing a Miller-Abbott tube. In the event of balloon rupture or leakage, mercury may produce a local inflammatory reaction when it lies free in the intestinal lumen. Acute appendicitis and small bowel fistulas have occurred as a direct result of mercury deposits within the lumen.

Finally, it should be restated that all patients with indwelling intestinal tubes suffer some impairment of respiratory drainage. For this reason, surgeons often prefer to perform a gastrostomy in older patients with respiratory disease after abdominal surgery rather than leave a tube within the pharynx, or in patients whose head-injury is severe enough to render them unconscious for long periods of time. Frequent coughing, humidity, positive pressure breathing, and other procedures designed to aid pulmonary drainage must be applied aggressively when tubes are in use. In addition, indwelling gastrointestinal tubes must not remain any longer than necessary! Prompt removal after their postoperative need has passed will often result in the disappearance of low grade fevers produced by retained secretions and pulmonary atelectasis.

### Selected References for Further Reading

1. Frank, H. A. and Green, L. C. Successful use of a bulk laxative to control the diarrhea of tube feeding. *Scand. J. Plast. Reconstr. Surg.* *13:*193–194, 1979.
2. Hafner, C. D., Wylie, J. H., and Brush, B. E. Complications of gastrointestinal intubation. *Arch. Surg. (Chicago) 83:* 147–160, 1961.
3. Machella, T. E. and Rhoads, J. E. Complications of gastrointestinal intubation. In *Complications in Surgery and Their Management,* edited by C. P. Artz and J. D. Hardy. W. B. Saunders, Philadelphia, 1960, pp. 622–638.
4. Miller, T. G. and Abbott, W. S. Intestinal intubation: a practical technique. *Amer. J. Med. Sci. 187:* 595–599, 1934.
5. Nealon, T. F. *Fundamental Skills in Surgery.* W. B. Saunders, Philadelphia, 1962, pp. 152–167.
6. Sengstaken, R. W. and Blakemore, A. H. Balloon tamponage for the control of hemorrhage from esophageal varices. *Ann. Surg. 131:* 781–789, 1950.

# FIFTEEN

# Sigmoidoscopy

Sigmoidoscopy is a simple yet valuable diagnostic technique which should be learned by all students with sufficient proficiency to cause minimal patient discomfort, yet permit careful examination of the last 25 cm of the lower intestine (where 70% of all colon and rectal disease occurs). Sigmoidoscopy should not be considered a difficult surgical procedure to be performed by specialists. Rather, it should be performed regularly on asymptomatic patients over 40 as a screen for early rectal and colonic disease.

## HISTORY

The invention of the sigmoidoscope closely paralleled the development of the cystoscope, since both devices depended on a satisfactory source of illumination. Phillip Rozzini has been credited as the inventor of the first endoscope (or "lichtleiter") which utilized a short candle as light source. In 1826, Pierre Segalas applied the endoscope principle for examination of the urethra and bladder. Modified versions of his instrument appeared in subsequent years with a number of light sources, ranging from petroleum and camphor candles to alcohol and turpentine lamps. An incandescent source of illumination was finally introduced by a German physician, Max Nitzl, in 1879.

Howard Kelly of The Johns Hopkins Hospital first advocated endoscope examination of the lower rectum as early as

1895, using light reflected from a head mirror as his source of illumination. In 1889, J. R. Pennington of Chicago succeeded in applying Nitzl's light source to the "Kelly tubes" and introduced an instrument most closely resembling the modern sigmoidoscope. Its use soon became widespread in this country, but not until 1905 was Pennington's sigmoidoscope introduced in Europe where most of the underlying principles upon which it was based originated.

## EQUIPMENT

A variety of sigmoidoscopes are available today but a lengthy discussion of their individual characteristics is not appropriate, since students and house staff rarely have the opportunity to select their own equipment. In brief, sigmoidoscopes are equipped with either proximal or distal lighting. Advocates of the former claim that the distal light becomes coated with residual bowel contents, whereas advocates of the latter like the brighter illumination which the distal bulb provides. The differences are subtle and the introduction of fiber optic sigmoidoscopes and illuminated disposable sigmoidoscopes should eliminate all cause for controversy.

It is worthwhile to define three terms often used synonymously: namely, proctoscopy, sigmoidoscopy, and protosigmoidoscopy. The final term is probably the most accurate but perhaps a bit cumbersome. A proctoscope is half the length of a sigmoidoscope and is designed for examination to the 12-cm level; it is not commonly used today. Its use, in fact, should be discouraged for, if a patient is to be subjected to endoscopy of any kind, it should be for the purpose of performing a full examination to the 25-cm level. In practice, the terms proctoscopy and sigmoidoscopy are often used interchangeably and ordinarily imply complete rectosigmoid examinations.

Another instrument which merits introduction is the anoscope, a short instrument with a beveled distal tip designed for use while examining the anal canal. The anoscope can be used in conjunction with a sigmoidoscope while performing a complete proctologic examination.

Most of the endoscopic instruments described above are of uniform diameter, 1.6 cm (¾ inch). Pediatric endoscopes are available but rarely necessary. Except for the infant, stool diameter in adults and children is almost equal, reflecting uniformity of anal sphincter tone. Therefore, most children are able to tolerate an adult scope without difficulty even though the examination might not extend to as high a level.

In addition to a sigmoidoscope, the examiner needs a satisfactory power source (often battery operated to allow portability). A suction device must be available with a tip of sufficient length. Other necessary items include an insufflation bag, a finger cot (or rubber gloves), lubricant, an anoscope, cotton-tipped swabs, biopsy forceps, and a specimen bottle. An electrocoagulation unit may also be helpful if a biopsy is to be done. Always remember to check all equipment to be certain it functions properly *before* positioning the patient or inserting the scope!

---

## NEEDED FOR SIGMOIDOSCOPY:

Disposable enema  
Finger cot or plastic glove  
Aqueous lubricant  
Anoscope  
Sigmoidoscope  
Light carrier  
Source of illumination  

Suction apparatus  
Insufflation bag  
Biopsy forceps  
Coagulation unit  
Specimen bottle  
Gauze pads or tissue  

---

## PREPARATION OF PATIENT

Opinions vary with respect to the need for special preparation of the rectum prior to examination. Some proctologists feel that three quarters of the ambulatory population may be examined satisfactorily without enemas. Preliminary irrigations, they feel, may aggravate pre-existent inflammatory conditions or wash away important clues, such as blood streaks. Others firmly recommend enema preps, in which case a single disposable enema of hypophosphate given 1–2 hours before examination is considered sufficient.

Regardless of one's individual prep philosophy, a sigmoidoscopic exam should not be postponed simply because a prep has not been done. Even if fecal material is encountered in the initial stages of the procedure, a temporary halt may be called until an enema can be administered.

Do not schedule sigmoidoscopy just prior to an intravenous pyelogram or barium enema since the radiologist's examination may be hindered by air insufflated during the procedure.

## POSITION OF PATIENT

Patients may be satisfactorily examined in one of several alternative positions. The prone or inverted position is most commonly used and may be accomplished either with a proctologic examination table or by having the patient assume a knee-chest position on a conventional examination table or bed. The primary advantage of this position is that the intestinal organs fall out of the pelvis, placing the distal sigmoid colon under some traction and facilitating the passing of the sigmoidoscope.

In this position, the patient's knees should be placed 6–8 inches apart in order to relax the gluteal musculature. Reassure the patient that he will neither fall forward nor sideways, and remember to preserve modesty by covering all but the anal region with a simple drape! At the completion of the procedure, advise patients to rise slowly. Stand by them a moment until they regain their balance in order to avoid fainting or a fall.

Elderly or seriously ill patients tolerate the knee-chest position poorly. In this instance, the lateral or Sims position may be used with ease in their own bed. After turning the patient on his side, the lower leg should be extended and the superior leg flexed at the knee and groin in order to spread the buttocks and lend stability to the position. If the buttocks extend over the edge of the bed 3–4 inches, this will facilitate a full arc for the scope. Many consider this preferable to all other sigmoidoscopy positions.

## TECHNIQUE

Make certain that all equipment is in good working order before beginning. After the patient is properly positioned and draped, begin to converse with him at his level of intelligence in order to relieve apprehension. Announce each new maneuver in advance, e.g. "You will now feel my gloved finger, which may feel cold." "I am now going to insert my finger into your rectum." "Please breathe deeply through your mouth." "I will now insert an instrument about the size of my finger and you will feel like you want to move your bowels," etc.

Observe the anal region carefully and make note of any inflammation, skin tags, or prolapsed hemorrhoid tissue. Look closely for fissures or abscesses which might declare themselves with sufficient pain to prevent further examination. Using a finger cot or rubber glove, proceed with a careful digital exam of the rectum. Use liberal quantities of lubricant. Nothing should be placed in the rectum without the aid of lubrication! Introduce the anoscope and examine all four quadrants, replacing the obturator each time before turning to the next area. Now take the sigmoidoscope with its obturator in place and apply lubricant. Aim the tip toward the patient's umbilicus as the sphincter is entered, advance the scope 2–3 cm, stop, remove the obturator, and insert the light carrier. Attach the insufflation bag for use at a later time if there is difficulty finding the lumen.

Now, under direct vision advance the scope slowly, *making certain that the lumen is visible ahead of the tip at all times*. As the rectum is entered, the direction of the scope will change as the tip follows the curve of the sacrum (Fig. 15.1). After the valves of Houston are passed, the mucosa loses its smooth character and circumferential rings appear, signifying entrance into the

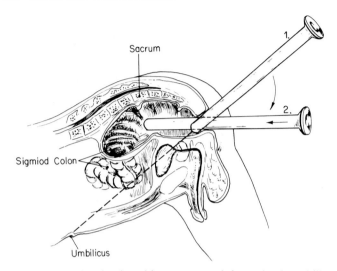

Sacrum

Sigmiod Colon

Umbilicus

**Figure 15.1.** Aim the sigmoidoscope toward the patient's umbilicus (1) as the spincter is entered and then shift the scope (2) and follow the curve of the sacrum until the sigmoid colon is reached.

sigmoid colon. The scope will usually advance to the 15-cm level with ease. At this point, the sigmoid colon curves to the patient's left and special care must be exercised. Patients may notice cramping pains if the mesentery is placed under excessive tension. Warn the patient of possible cramps at this point. Occasionally, the mesentery is short and the scope will not negotiate the rather sharp bend, even in the most experienced hands. In this instance, terminate further advancement. Above all, *do not hurt the patient*!

Ordinarily, the sigmoidoscope will pass to the 25-cm level without difficulty in 60–70% of cases. At this point, insufflation or air may allow the examiner to see another 1–5 cm ahead of the scope. Although insufflation is designed to allow distention of the bowel through the examination, its use should be limited since excessive air may be traumatic and painful.

After advancing the scope as far as possible, tell the patient that the procedure is nearly complete and that little or no discomfort should be experienced during withdrawal. However, it is at this point that the examination begins in earnest. All attention during advancement of the scope should be directed toward a safe and painless passage, whereas the most careful scrutiny of the bowel for pathologic conditions is carried out during withdrawal. Pull back slowly using a small rotatory motion in order to view all mucosal surfaces. This is most essential in the rectum, where the lumen diameter is larger and the posterior surface coursing over the sacral convexity is not always in view. Flatten each rectal valve ridge with the tip of the scope in order not to miss lesions on their proximal surface. Always remember to release any air placed in the sigmoid just prior to removing the sigmoidoscope or else cramps may persist. Finally, remember to remove residual lubricant from the buttocks with a tissue before the patient departs.

If the examination has revealed nothing abnormal, be certain to tell the patient so. Don't limit yourself to indefinite terminology, such as growth, tumor, polyp, etc. Patients want to know that they *do not have cancer*! If there have been positive findings, it is wise to defer specific comments, stating that necessary biopsies will require time for microscopic study.

## RECTAL BIOPSY AND POLYPECTOMY

All observed lesions should be biopsied promptly in order to prevent a delay in diagnosis. Therefore, sigmoidoscopy should not be performed in the absence of biopsy equipment. Polypectomy, on the other hand, is often deferred until after a barium enema, since there is danger of perforation if the order is reversed.

A simple rectal biopsy forceps is adequate for taking small specimens at the tip or the most suspicious area of a lesion. Bleeding is ordinarily minimal and may be controlled with pressure exerted by a cotton-tipped swab. However, a snare is necessary to remove large polyps and this is best done in the operating room under optimal conditions, particularly if the lesion resides above the level of the peritoneal reflection (more than 12 cm). Bleeding may be more vigorous at the base of a polyp; therefore, an electrocoagulation must be available.

Remember to label specimens separately and according to level—particularly when more than one has been removed. The discovery of malignancy in one of several specimens removed from different sites, but sent to the pathology department in the same bottle, is unfortunate for patient and physician alike.

# COMPLICATIONS

Crampy pains and low grade fever may occasionally follow sigmoidoscopy. This may be due to mild peritoneal irritation or excessive introduction of air, but it is ordinarily transient. Hemorrhage, as has already been mentioned briefly, may be vigorous following polypectomy and requires cautery of the stalk. If care is not taken to obtain hemostasis at the time of surgery, then a bloody bowel movement may occur several hours later and necessitate a revisit to the operating room.

Perforation of the bowel undoubtedly represents the most serious complication of sigmoidoscopy, since it necessitates prompt surgical exploration! This most commonly occurs on the antimesenteric border at about 15 cm, where the sigmoid takes its first sharp turn. The event is usually quite obvious since bleeding occurs and peritoneal fluid, small bowel, and omentum may be visualized ahead of the sigmoidoscope. The cause is almost always related to excessive force being applied at a time when the lumen cannot be visualized ahead of the scope!

In the event of perforation into the peritoneum, prompt recognition is absolutely essential, since laparotomy and closure will usually prevent any serious consequences of the deed. However, any delay in recognition will necessitate a colostomy and further increase morbidity, in addition to risking the patient's life.

Perforations may also occur in the rectum in which case the scope enters the retroperitoneal space. This has resulted not only from sigmoidoscopy but also following careless administration of enemas. Low perforation is heralded by fever and evidenced radigraphically by retroperitoneal emphysema, i.e. air shadows along the psoas shadows. Treatment is usually conservative, although pararectal abscesses may develop and require drainage at a later time. Remember that perforations are almost always a result of force and can be prevented by good visibility and a gentle hand.

### Selected References for Further Reading

1. Harley, P. H. and Hines, M. O. Analysis of two thousand consecutive proctologic examinations. *Southern Med. J. 49:* 475–484, 1956.
2. Moertel, C. G., Hill, J. R., and Dockerty, M. B. The routine protoscopic examination. *Mayo Clin. Proc. 41:* 368–874, 1966.
3. Nesselrod, J. P. *Clinical Proctology*, 3rd Ed. W. B. Saunders, Philadelphia, 1964.

# SIXTEEN

# Paracentesis

Paracentesis or abdominal tap may be utilized either for diagnostic or for therapeutic reasons. The aspiration of blood-stained peritoneal fluid or any serous fluid containing elevated amylase levels is clinically significant. Peritoneal lavage and culdocentesis are useful variations of this technique. Cirrhotics with massive ascites breathe better after removal of excess abdominal fluid. Yet another application is peritoneal dialysis which involves the insertion of a specially designed trocar through which large volumes of fluid are infused and collected. Less commonly performed today is pneumoperitoneum, i.e. the introduction of air into the peritoneal cavity for the treatment of tuberculosis. Perhaps the only reason that air might be introduced today is for radiological procedures designed to demonstrate enlarged organs (e.g. adrenal tumors). This chapter considers only the first two indications, namely diagnostic abdominal tap (and lavage) and therapeutic paracentesis for the removal of ascitic fluid.

## POSITION

The position of the patient depends upon the procedure to be done. Patients tolerate a sitting position more easily whenever excessive fluid interferes with respiration (Fig. 16.1). If the procedure is for diagnostic procedures only, the patient may be more comfortable lying down. If culdocentesis is to be

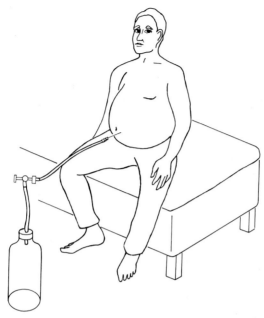

**Figure 16.1.**   Therapeutic paracentesis with position of patient and drainage technique.

performed, the patient must be placed in a lithotomy position (Fig. 18.1).

## EQUIPMENT

Essential for a diagnostic tap are the following: a local anesthetic, a syringe, a 20-gauge long needle with a short bevel, and a No. 11 scalpel blade. Peritoneal lavage will require in addition: a trocar, a peritoneal dialysis catheter, and one liter of normal saline. An over needle catheter or through needle catheter may be substituted. Culdocentesis will require a vaginal speculum, a cervical tenaculum, and a long sponge forceps. Either a needle or trocar may be selected for removing ascitic fluid, transabdominally. Ascitic fluid can be drawn efficiently into vacuum sealed bottles. If none are available, then a 50-ml syringe is a satisfactory substitute.

# TECHNIQUE

The site for both paracentesis and peritoneal lavage is in the midline just beneath the umbilicus, perhaps because this region can distend more with fluid, particularly when the patient rests in a sitting position. The area is relatively thin, devoid of large blood vessels that might be punctured and there is generally less preperitoneal fat. Old surgical scars must be avoided for they might be cause for adherent bowel. Perforation of the bowel might result, therefore, following needle insertion (Fig. 16.2). If the patient has had extensive pelvic surgery, it might be well to select the upper abdomen. Always ask the patient to void prior to the procedure so that a bladder distended with urine will not interrupt your purpose. A gravid uterus is always a contraindication to lower abdominal tap or lavage.

# DIAGNOSTIC TAP

After identifying the site, prepare the skin with an antiseptic, anesthetize a small zone with 1% Lidocaine, and pierce the skin with a tip of a No. 11 scalpel blade. Using a short bevel 20-gauge needle and a 10-ml syringe, advance to the level of the fascia. Apply gentle pressure until there is a sudden release of resistance (as the needle pierces the peritoneum). Nonadherent bowel is normally pushed away by the needle and rarely punctured unless adhesions are present. Collect a sample of peritoneal fluid and carefully note its color. If bloody or bile stained fluid, urine, or feces return, an appropriate diagnosis can be made. Negative taps, on the other hand, do not indicate absence of hemorrhage or of ruptured viscous.

## Peritoneal Lavage

Peritoneal lavage represents a technique for more sensitive detection of intra-abdominal injury following blunt abdominal

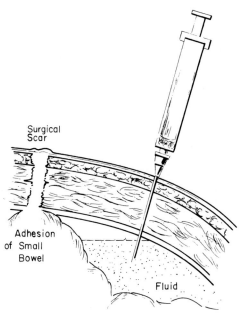

**Figure 16.2.** Surgical incision sites must be avoided since they are often associated with intestinal adhesions, and perforation may result from paracentesis carried out nearby.

trauma. It permits the surgeon to discover intra-abdominal bleeding at an earlier phase, often before there is clinical evidence of shock or hemoperitoneum. It is used whenever physical findings are equivocal for intra-abdominal injury or when the physical examination is unreliable, perhaps because the patient is comatose, or exhibits a neurological deficit. Peritoneal lavage may be used in patients with multiple-system trauma requiring emergency surgery or other circumstances when it would be tragic to have overlooked an intra-abdominal hemorrhage, such as during anesthesia. Peritoneal lavage is not indicated in the case of penetrating wounds of the abdomen because these are usually explored surgically or where free blood in the abdomen is not particularly helpful diagnostically (pelvic fractures). The other contraindications are similar to those for a paracentesis.

Lavage is accomplished by insertion of a dialysis catheter through a trocar placed into the lower abdomen (Fig. 16.3), or it may be done using a through the needle catheter (16-gauge). Abdominal skin is first prepared with antiseptic and the skin is anesthetized about 2 cm below the umbilicus in the midline and infiltrated down to the fascia with 1% Lidocaine and epinephrine. A 2-cm incision is made and the midline fascia is exposed (Fig. 16.3A). Perfect hemostasis must be established before continuing to avoid contamination of the field with blood. One milliliter of anesthetic agent with epinephrine is injected through the fascia. Nick the fascia with a scalpel and insert the trocar into the peritoneal cavity directing it toward the patient's sacrum (Fig. 16.3B). Once the tip lies just within the peritoneal cavity, a dialysis catheter is introduced through the trocar and the trocar is withdrawn. Aspiration is attempted

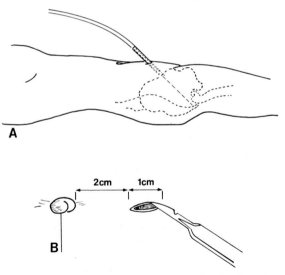

**Figure 16.3.** Placement of dialysis catheter, showing location of the incision (B) and insertion angle of the trocar and dialysis catheter (A).

then with a positive diagnosis being similar to that of paracentesis, but, if the aspiration is negative, the catheter is attached
to an infusion system (15 ml/kg) over the next 20 minutes.
While there is still fluid present in the tubing, the infusion
bottle is placed on the floor and the infused fluid is siphoned
out (Fig. 16.4). The returned fluid is examined for red blood
cells, white blood cells, bile, amylase, and sometimes culture
and antibiotic sensitivity. Table 16.1 lists all possible findings
and their corresponding appropriate interpretation. After as
much fluid as possible has been siphoned from the abdominal
cavity, the catheter is withdrawn and the skin is closed with
interrupted 4-0 nylon sutures. This method is far more sensitive
than a simple tap and will more reliably detect intraperitoneal
hemorrhage not yet evident.

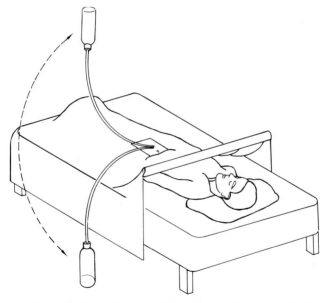

**Figure 16.4.**  Peritoneal lavage. After all the fluid has drained into
the abdomen, lower the bottle to siphon out the fluid.

**Table 16.1.   Interpretation of Results of Diagnostic Peritoneal Lavage**

|  | Test Result |
|---|---|
| Blood in catheter | Positive |
| Aspiration of blood, bile, urine, or feces | Positive |
| Clear or pink fluid | Negative* |
| Grossly bloody lavage fluid | Positive |
| Many red blood cells in lavage fluid |  |
| (>100,000 RBC/ml) | Positive |
| (>50,000 RBC/ml) | Suspicious |
| Many white blood cells in lavage fluid |  |
| (>500 WBC/ml) | Positive |
| (>100 WBC/ml) | Suspicious |
| Bile or intestinal contents in lavage fluid | Positive |
| Bacteria in lavage fluid | Positive |
| High amylase activity |  |
| (>175 $\mu$/dl) | Positive |
| (>75 $\mu$/dl) | Suspicious |

* Presumed negative pending microscopic study.

## Culdocentesis

Culdocentesis is a technique that is especially useful for detecting ectopic pregnancy. It might also be substituted for peritoneal lavage among women suspected of sustaining occult trauma. The cul-de-sac is the most dependent portion of the peritoneal cavity. Bleeding anywhere within the peritoneal cavity will produce at least a small collection of blood within the cul-de-sac. Culdocentesis is performed by placing a speculum into the vagina and clearly visualizing the cervix. Lift the cervix with a cervical tenaculum or sponge forceps and insert a long No. 18-gauge needle into the cul-de-sac immediately posterior to the cervix, taking care to avoid injury to the rectum. Aspiration of blood or blood-stained peritoneal fluid is diagnostic. The primary risk of culdocentesis is damage to adjacent structures. It is contraindicated after pelvic surgery because of the likelihood that loops of bowel will be adhered to the cul-de-sac.

## Therapeutic Tap

Prepare the skin and introduce either a needle or trocar as described under diagnostic tap (Fig. 16.1). Then attach the needle or catheter to a vacuum bottle with plastic intravenous tubing. Limit aspiration to 1000 of ascitic fluid at one time. Avoid removing larger volumes since rapid fluid shifts might occur, leading to hemoconcentration and hypovolemia in some cases. It is far safer to perform multiple taps on successive or alternate days than to drain the entire volume at one time.

# COMPLICATIONS

The risk of bladder, uterus, and bowel perforation have already been described together with the means to prevent each potential injury. When inadvertent viscous puncture occurs, withdraw the needle and try again in another site. Such complications are ordinarily not very serious. Puncture with a trocar might produce a more serious injury requiring exploration and repair, but certainly not always. Persistent leakage of ascitic fluid through the puncture site is uncommon, but is managed successfully in most instances by placing a suture in the skin aperture. Multiple needle aspirations in various locations of the abdomen, such as the so-called four quadrant tap, may make the abdomen somewhat tender and interfere with subsequent examination for abdominal tenderness. Abdominal wall hematomas following paracentesis might cause the examiner to make false interpretations or else confuse future abdominal examinations.

### Selected References for Further Reading

1. Ahmad, W. and Polk, H. C., Jr. Blunt abdominal trauma: a study of relationship between diagnosis and outcome. *Southern Med. J. 66:* 1127–1130, 1973.
2. Bivins, B. A., Jonas, J. Z., and Belm, R. P. Diagnostic peritoneal lavage in pediatric trauma. *J. Trauma 16:* 739–742, 1976.
3. Drapanas, T. and McDonald, J. Peritoneal tap in abdominal trauma. *Surgery 100:* 22, 1960.
4. Drew, R., Perry, J. F., and Fischer, R. P. The expediency of peritoneal lavage for blunt trauma in children. *Surg. Gynec. Obstet. 145:* 885–888, 1977.

5. Fischer, R. P., Beuerlin, B. C., Engrav, L. H., Benjamin, C. I., and Perry, J. F. Diagnostic peritoneal lavage: fourteen years and 2,586 patients later. *Amer. J. Surg. 136:* 701–704, 1978.

6. Moretz, W. H. and Erickson, W. G. Peritoneal tap as an aide in the diagnosis of acute abdominal disease. *Amer. Surg. 20:* 363, 1954.

7. Olsen, W. R., Redman, H. C., and Hildreth, D. H. Quantitative peritoneal lavage in blunt abdominal trauma. *Ann. Surg. 104:* 536–543, 1972.

8. Parvin, S., Smith, D. E., Osher, W. M., and Virgilio, R. W. Effectiveness of peritoneal lavage in blunt abdominal trauma. *Ann. Surg. 181:* 255–262, 1975.

9. Perry, J. F., Jr. Blunt and penetrating abdominal injuries. In *Current Problems in Surgery.* Yearbook Medical Publishers, Inc., Chicago, 1970.

10. Powell, R. W., Smith, D. E., Zarins, C. K., Parvin, S., and Virgilio, R. W. Peritoneal lavage in children with blunt abdominal trauma. *J. Pediat. Surg. 11:* 973–977, 1976.

11. Root, H. D., Hauser, C. S., McKinley, C. R., LaFave, J. W., and Mendiola, R. P., Jr. Diagnostic peritoneal lavage. *Surgery 57:* 633–637, 1965.

12. Strickler, J. H., Erwin, T. D., and Rice, C. O. Diagnostic paracentesis. *Arch. Surg. 77:* 859–863, 1958.

# SEVENTEEN

# Urethral Catheterization

Catheters are introduced into the urinary bladder for one or more of the following reasons: 1) to obtain a urine specimen for routine analysis or culture, 2) to confirm the presence of and measure residual urine, 3) to relieve acute urinary retention, 4) to provide continuous bladder drainage, or 5) monitor urinary output. This chapter discusses simple catheterization as it pertains to all of the above indications but omits special instrumentation techniques which are considered in detail in many urologic textbooks.

## HISTORY

Although the origins of urologic instruments go back to ancient times, the flexible catheter is a relatively modern invention. The Egyptians used metal sounds as early as 3000 B.C., and Susruta, the great Hindu physician, described dilators, probes, sounds, and stone forceps made of wood, iron, or gold. The Chinese made what was perhaps the first true catheter out of a tubular rolled leaf to which several coats of lacquer were applied. All of these early devices shared one common feature—they were perfectly straight since their inventors paid no heed to the anatomy of the posterior urethra.

Galen constructed the first S-shaped catheter. Avicenna introduced the first flexible catheter in 1036 A.D. The 19th century witnessed the introduction of a number of elastic woven catheters, one of which, the Coude catheter, is still used today.

Two events contributed to the development of the urethral catheter as we know it. First, a French surgeon named Nelaton constructed a soft red rubber catheter and, second, Charles Goodyear learned how to vulcanize rubber. Nelaton saw Goodyear's display at the London Exhibition of 1851 and adapted the process for his own invention.

For the next several decades, rubber catheters underwent minor refinements, but in 1927, Dr. Theodore Davis of Greenville, South Carolina, thought of adding inflatable balloons to the end of catheters so that hemorrhage following prostatic resection could be controlled through tamponade. Somehow the idea never advanced beyond the drawing board until Dr. F.E.B. Foley of St. Paul, Minnesota succeeded in constructing such a device and convinced the C. R. Bard Company to manufacture it commercially. His invention is still widely used today, although it is more frequently applied as a self-retaining catheter than for the control of hemorrhage.

# EQUIPMENT

Catheters are selected according to the use for which they are intended. Two major varieties are available: 1) the simple, straight, nonretention catheter, and 2) the self-retaining balloon catheter. The first is suitable for short-term insertion in order to obtain specimens or to relieve acute bladder distention. The Foley balloon catheter is the most common variety of self-retaining device and is designed to be left in place for long-term drainage. A modification of the Foley is the three-way catheter, which incorporates an additional lumen for the purpose of irrigating the bladder. Both simple and self-retaining catheters are available with semi-rigid tips. The most popular of these is the Coude catheter, which is helpful in patients with prostatic hypertrophy because its curved and rigid tip will pass through the angulated prostatic urethra. However, it should be used only under the supervision of a urologist who is thoroughly familiar with instrumentation of the urethra.

Most urethral catheters are constructed of soft rubber. Siliconized rubber and several plastics have been employed recently in the construction of catheters resulting in less tissue reaction (urethritis). Glass catheters, once popular in Great Britain, should now be avoided altogether.

Calibration of catheter diameter is a confusing topic. According to the French scale, each gradation equals one-third of a millimeter. Therefore, an 18 French catheter has a diameter of 6 mm. There are also American (A) and English (E) scales with each gradation equal to 0.5 mm, but the English scale is two numbers behind the American. Therefore, 10 mm = 30 Fr = 20 A = 18 E. The French scale is used most commonly.

The size of catheter used will depend upon several factors: among them age, sex, and intended purpose. For the adult, large diameters (16–22 Fr) are easier to introduce and less traumatic to the urethra. Narrow catheters (10–14 Fr) are suitable for children but should be avoided in adults, since they lack stiffness and tend to coil within the urethra when the tip reaches the external sphincter. In the absence of stricture, the external meatus is the narrowest part of the normal urethra, so that catheters passing that point will ordinarily go the rest of the way.

Smaller catheters may be used in women. Special care is necessary when children are involved. The urethra of a 6-year-old female will ordinarily admit a 12 Fr catheter, but a boy will take only 10 Fr. Infants require even narrower catheters.

---

## NEEDED FOR CATHETERIZING A BLADDER:

Disposable catheterization tray (includes some but not all of the following):

Prep sponges and solution (e.g. Povidone-iodine)

Foley or straight catheter

Aqueous lubricant

Sterile gloves

Clamp

Sterile closed drainage bag

Specimen bottle

Foley catheters available today come with 5- and 30-cc inflatable balloons. The smaller balloons are most often selected, but the 30-cc balloon is useful for postoperative patients following transurethral resection of the prostate. Many urologists recommend the use of 30-cc balloons in confused patients, provided that they are inflated with only 20 cc of water. The catheter will be difficult to dislodge, but forceful removal will not result in nearly the degree of urethral injury that a fully inflated 30-cc bag will produce.

Other equipment used for urethral catheterization includes sterile gloves, a small metal basin, and a glass specimen bottle for urine collection, draping sheets, sponges, prep solution, *aqueous* lubricant, a 10-cc syringe, forceps or hemostatic clamp, and a catheter clamp.

## TECHNIQUE

The importance of aseptic technique cannot be over emphasized. A catheter cannot be passed with complete sterility because of the bacteria which normally reside within the distal urethra. But since infection remains the most common complication of catheterization, all efforts should be directed toward the limitation of bacterial contamination.

Begin by checking the assembled equipment while explaining the procedure to the patient. The legs should be slightly abducted. Position the tray of equipment near the bed and open it before donning sterile gloves. Do not place the tray on or between the patient's legs since unexpected patient movement may send everything tumbling to the floor. If a Foley catheter is to be used, draw saline into a syringe and inflate the balloon to test for leaks, then deflate the balloon and set the filled syringe nearby, where it can be reached easily later.

When catheterizing men, place sterile towels around the base of the penis. The shaft may even be held with a drape in a way that the glove is not contaminated. A drape should also be placed inferior to the penis. Cleanse the glans gently with an appropriate solution (e.g. Povidone-iodine). Alcohol or other astringent solutions should never be used. pHisoHex is also a poor choice since it is irritating to scrotal skin. If the patient has not been circumcized, retract the foreskin before prepping. The accumulated smegma beneath the foreskin is a favorite breeding ground for bacteria of all kinds, as well as for non-pathogenic acid-fast bacilli.

Lubricate the catheter very well prior to insertion—not just the tip but the distal 6–10 cm. A favorite method of urologists involves injection of 10–15 cc of lubricant into the urethra with a glass-tipped bulb syringe.

Now, if one hand is still holding the penis and the other has been used for the prep, then no sterile hand is available to pass the catheter. Therefore, introduce the catheter with a hemo-static clamp (Fig. 17.1). By holding the penis at right angles to the axis of the body, the urethra is converted from an S-curve into a gentle C. Advance the catheter slowly but firmly. In the absence of a stricture, the catheter should pass easily until the tip reaches the external bladder sphincter. Resistance at this point is due to involuntary muscle spasm which can be avoided

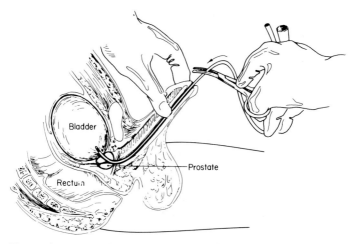

**Figure 17.1.** Extend the penis and insert the well lubricated catheter slowly with a Kelly clamp.

by asking the patient to take a deep breath and relax as much as possible.

If a straight catheter is being used, advance it only until urine returns. A Foley catheter, however, should be inserted as far as possible before the balloon is inflated, and then withdrawn until resistance is felt as the balloon abuts the bladder neck. This precaution will avoid the error of inflating the balloon while it lies within the prostatic urethra. Finally, collect a urine specimen before connecting the catheter (if it is to remain) to a sterile closed drainage collection apparatus.

Catheterization of women is far simpler since the female urethra is only 3–4 cm long. Nevertheless, a few technical points should be observed. A woman must be in the lithotomy position for catheterization (that is, with knees flexed and thighs abducted, see Fig. 18.1). With the finger and thumb of one hand, spread the labia apart maximally, so that the entire vulvar area can be seen. When the area is free of genital hair, the other hand may be used for cleansing and catheterizing, as in the case of the male. It should be emphasized that, if the labia are not spread and the urethral meatus observed directly, two problems might arise: 1) the risk of carrying vulvar pathogens into the bladder with the catheter, or 2) the potential for the catheter to follow the path of least resistance and enter the vagina instead of the bladder!

## SPECIAL PROBLEMS

### Maintenance of Catheter Drainage

The prevention of early bacterial contamination depends upon a sterile, closed urine collecting system (Fig. 17.2). A number of tubing sets are available which connect indwelling catheters to expandable plastic receptacles. There should be sufficient play in the collection tubing so that the catheter will not be dislodged or placed on tension when the patient turns over. Securing the tubing to the patient's thigh or abdomen with adhesive tape is helpful. Ideally, the collection apparatus should remain closed until the catheter is removed or changed.

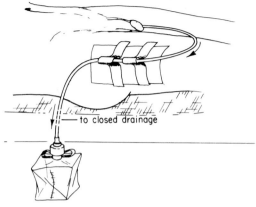

— to closed drainage

**Figure 17.2.**  Always use closed drainage and secure the tubing to the abdomen or the leg.

However, the catheter must be separated from the tubing if irrigation becomes necessary to remove blood clots or deposits. Gloves should be worn and extra care should be taken to avoid outside contamination whenever this is done. Catheters require frequent irrigation (20–30 cc of sterile saline) whenever the urine contains blood clots or whenever drainage is insufficient. The urine receptacle should never be raised higher than the catheter or contaminated urine may reflux into the bladder.

Catheter changes are indicated whenever obstruction cannot be relieved by irrigation. Frequent changes are inadvisable since each new catheter insertion carries an added risk of bacterial contamination.

### Prostatic Obstruction

Catheterization of the patient with prostatic hypertrophy may be exceedingly difficult. If the catheter meets obstruction at the bladder neck, one of the following measures may bring success: 1) fill the urethra with 10–15 cc of lubricant with a glass-tipped syringe and then try again. 2) Try a smaller catheter. If this also fails, then try a larger caliber which has increased rigidity. 3) Turn the patient on his side, and with a gloved finger in the rectum attempt to guide the catheter tip *gently* past the obstruction.

If success has not been achieved, final recourse lies with the use of either a stylet or curved tip (Coude) catheter. The employment of these devices, however, should only be done by or under the supervision of a physician trained in urology.

### Measuring Residual Urine

Residual urine may be defined as that volume which resides within the bladder immediately after the patient has voided. Normally, in the well compensated bladder, this volume is less than 10 cc. Measurement is made by passing a catheter soon after the patient has voided.

### Decompression of the Chronically Distended Bladder

Patients with prostatic hypertrophy may slowly accumulate a large volume of urine (as much as 2,000–2,500 cc), even though they void small amounts each day. If this goes unrecognized, uremia will develop. Complications have been reported when such a bladder is quickly decompressed. Urologists used to speak of "catastrophic catheterization," meaning renal failure and death following bladder decompression. It is now recognized that anuria develops prior to catheterization, probably a combined result of obstructive uropathy and infection.

### Penile Obstruction

Any obstruction encountered other than at the bladder neck probably represents a pre-existent stricture. Ask the patient whether he has previously required dilation. Persistent attempts to traverse the area without dilation will result in urethral trauma and might worsen the stricture!

## COMPLICATIONS

1. Infection stands as the most common and potentially dangerous result of urethral catheterization. Kass noted that

2–3% of patients will develop urinary tract infections after a single catheterization. If the catheter remains indwelling, this figure rises rapidly with each passing day. Studies have shown that, after 4–7 days, significant bacilluria may be found in 95% of patients with indwelling catheters.

Many attempts have been made to improve these statistics. Measures such as aseptic technique during catheter insertion, strict maintenance of a closed drainage system, and application of topical antibiotic ointment to the urethral meatus have all been of some help in minimizing infection. Opinions vary on the use of systemic prophylactic antibiotics (e.g. Nitrofurantoin), since no clinical study has conclusively demonstrated their advantage.

2. Stricture may result from traumatic catheter insertion, use of caustic agents in the urethra, or prolonged use of catheters which produce erosions of the urethral mucosa and urethritis. Generally, the larger catheters are more likely to produce urethritis, since they impede the escape of urethral secretions. Similarly, in the male, a large bore catheter may obstruct prostatic and vesicular secretions or else lead to the development of epididymitis.

3. Fat embolism has been reported following forceful injection of lubricants into the urethra. Only aqueous lubricants should be used, and force must be avoided, particularly when patients have just experienced prostatic resection.

4. The undeflatable balloon is fortunately a rare problem today because of the excellence of manufacturing methods. It does, however, occur infrequently and can be a distressing problem to the physician. Several methods are available to overcome this predicament, among them deliberate overdistention of the balloon with saline until it bursts, or infusion of mineral oil into the balloon to allow deflation. When a balloon has burst in the bladder, careful inspection of the fragmented balloon should be made when the catheter is removed, because a retained foreign body in the bladder can lead to calculus formation.

One particularly unusual experience has been reported in which a balloon resisted all deflation efforts and finally separated from the catheter and remained inside floating about the bladder freely. Cystoscopy and attempted coagulation of the balloon failed and a suprapubic cystotomy was required to remove it. Hopefully, few physicians will experience as difficult and unusual a complication as this, but it is illustrative of how reliance upon man-made devices can have serious consequences.

### Selected References for Further Reading

1. Ansell, J. Some observations on catheter care. *J. Chronic Dis. 15:* 675–682, 1962.
2. Beeson, P. B. The case against the catheter. *Amer. J. Med. 24:* 1–3, 1958.
3. Kass, E. H. and Schneiderman, J. J. Entry of bacteria into the urinary tracts of patients with inlying catheters. *New Eng. J. Med. 256:* 556–557, 1957.
4. Kass, E. H. and Sossen, H. S. Prevention of infection of urinary tract in presence of indwelling catheters. *J.A.M.A. 169:* 1181–1183, 1959.
5. Turck, M. and Petersdorf, R. G. The role of antibiotics in the prevention of urinary tract infections. *J. Chronic Dis. 15:* 683–689, 1962.

# EIGHTEEN

# Pelvic Examination

Each patient seeking medical attention for complaints presumably pelvic in origin should first receive a complete history and physical examination. Only in this way will other diseases, such as cancer of the breast, heart disease, and other conditions, be discovered in their earlier stages. The pelvic and rectal examinations are important parts of the complete physical examination and it behooves practitioners of medicine to become an "expert" in the art and skill of pelvic examination for the benefit of all women who seek medical attention from a wide variety of medical specialists. To "defer" the pelvic examination implies that the patient has, in fact, not been examined.

## HISTORY

The art and practice of gynecology dates back to the time of the ancient Egyptians, the old Testament, and the early Greeks. Superstition and folklore have clouded much of female physiology until modern times and fantasies surrounding human reproduction persist even into this century.

Modern gynecological surgery dates from 1809 when Dr. Ephraim McDowell of Danville, Kentucky performed the first ovariotomy for a large ovarian cyst. Langenbeck reported the first vaginal hysterectomy in 1817. Sims described successful closure of a vesicovaginal fistula in 1852. Many others have contributed to the advancement of gynecology, but perhaps none so dramatically as Papanicolaou and Trant's classic work on vaginal cytology for cancer screening. These accomplishments have been utilized by many practitioners for the good of womankind.

## PREPARATION OF THE PATIENT

Most women dislike a pelvic examination and present for examination with much reservation. Privacy, dignity, and gentleness are essential. It is important that both the patient and the examiner be comfortable and that the examination be performed gently. A brief preparatory interview affords opportunity to explain the purpose of the exam, describe the procedure to the patient, thus assuring her confidence and relaxation. If the patient remains tense and frightened, the information gained from the examination will be limited. In spite of present regard for sexuality, a vast number of women have never had a pelvic examination or, if one has been performed, it was done nonchalantly with total disregard to the patient's apprehension. The first pelvic examination sets the tone for all future exams and, with explanation, will be accepted as one not to be feared.

## POSITION

Before being placed on the examining table, the patient should be asked to empty her urinary bladder and disrobe. If an unduly long period transpires from the time the patient first voided to the time of the pelvic exam, the bladder may refill. Many a "cyst" was merely a bladder with 200 ml of urine! In this same reasoning, firm pelvic masses may be merely constipated stool in the sigmoid colon and occasionally this differential must be learned, for the mass disappears with an enema! The female assistant puts the patient in position and drapes her for a pelvic examination. Routine pelvic examinations are done with the woman in the lithotomy position with the legs placed in stirrups (Fig. 18.1). In special cases, the Sims position (lateral prone position), the knee-chest position, or the standing position may be used. The knee-chest position is excellent for complete examination of the vaginal walls and for rectal examination in the adult and in young children since the filling of the vault with air acts as a natural dilator. Neither the Sims position nor the knee-chest position are as satisfactory for bimanual palpation.

## EQUIPMENT

The examiner is seated on a stool facing the patient's perineum. An instrument table equipped with the necessary supplies is within easy reach. The perineum is brightly illuminated either by a goosenecked lamp placed behind the examiner or by one of the several varieties of available headlights. An ordinary flashlight can provide excellent illumination for the whole procedure, but has the disadvantage of immobilizing one of the examiner's hands.

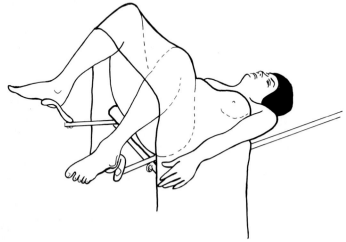

**Figure 18.1.** Lithotomy position.

## NEEDED FOR A PELVIC EXAM:

| | |
|---|---|
| Light | Fixative for cytology smears |
| Examining gloves | Surgical lubricant |
| Vaginal speculums, assorted sizes | Culture tubes |
| Nasal speculum | Biopsy forceps |
| Glass slides | Cotton swabs |
| Cervical spatula | Aqueous iodine solution |
| Aspirating tubes | Long pickup forceps |
| | Uterine probes |

## TECHNIQUE

The examiner wears a rubber glove on the hand used for digital examination (usually the left hand, but some prefer the dominant hand). Inspection of the external genitalia is made and their configuration and development are noted. One looks for evidence of infection, neoplasia, hypertrophy, atrophy, or trauma. The character and distribution of the pubic hair, texture of the skin, location of scars, sinus openings, and hemorrhoids are noted. The patient is first warned ("Now I am going to touch you" or "Now I am going to spread the lips of your vagina") and then the labia are separated by the thumb and forefinger of the gloved hand and the vestibule inspected (Fig. 18.2). The size and shape of the clitoris is noted. The presence or absence of discharge from the urethral orifice and the size, color, and configuration of the orifice are determined. The vaginal outlet (introitus) is inspected for discharge and Skene's glands and Bartholin's glands are palpated. The hymen is inspected and may be described as imperforate, virginal, or marital. If the hymen is perforate, tell the patient that you will place a finger into the vagina and then do so very gently. This prepares even the virgin for the actual instrument since she can "become used to" the dilating finger first.

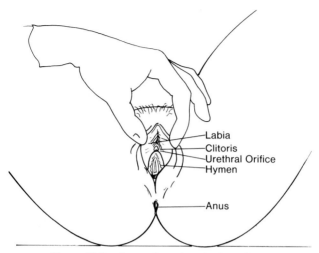

**Figure 18.2.** Inspection of vaginal vestibule.

The speculum examination follows (Fig. 18.3). The bivalve speculum should be at approximately body temperature, sterile, and suitably sized. If the patient complains of leukorrhea, do not place a lubricating material on the speculum blades since the lubricant will immobilize trichomonads and prevent the diagnosis of *Trichomanas vaginalis* vaginitis as a cause for the leukorrhea. If no leukorrhea is present, place the lubricant on the outer surfaces of the anterior and posterior blades of the speculum. The instrument is held in the right hand while the gloved left hand separates the labia. With a finger in the vagina, exert gentle downward pressure and instruct the patient to "relax these muscles." This will allow maximum space for the speculum. The speculum is introduced with the blades closed into the full length of the vagina using slight pressure against the posterior vaginal wall at a 45° angle to conform with its normal axis. The blades are opened and the cervix exposed.

Inspect the vaginal walls for infection, atrophy, trauma, bleeding, and tumors. The amount, color, and character of the

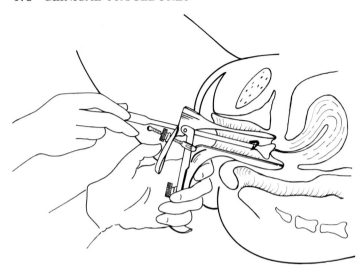

**Figure 18.3.** Diagram of the proper position of the speculum for inspection of the cervix uteri. A spatula is rotated in the cervical os to obtain cells for Pap smear.

discharge are noted. Bacteriological specimens may be taken from the vagina or cervix. Smears or hanging drops may be made also.

The size and condition of the cervix are noted as well as the size and shape of the cervical os. The presence of nabothian glands, tumors, polyps, cysts, infection, or trauma is determined. A Papanicolaou vaginal cytology test may be done at the initial pelvic examination unless bleeding is present. Material for direct smears for cytological study is obtained by scraping the exposed cervical os with a cervical specimen spatula (Fig. 18.3). Lesions on the cervix are more easily identified by using the Schiller's iodine solution to define the normal mahogany brown epithelium from the unstained diseased areas. Suspicious areas can be evaluated by vaginal microscopy or biopsy.

The digital examination of the introitus and vagina is made next. Two fingers of the gloved hand are placed against the posterior vaginal wall and perineal body thus depressing the perineal body. The patient is asked to cough. Many times a spurt of urine is forced out the urethral opening or a pouching of the urethra occurs below this orifice (urethrocele). Relaxation of the anterior vaginal wall (cystocele) can be demonstrated in a similar manner. The patient may be examined for rectocele by elevating the anterior vaginal wall with the gloved fingers and asking the patient to "bear down." This causes a bulging forward of the rectum against the posterior vaginal wall.

The examiner proceeds to the bimanual part of the examination and usually stands for this procedure. The lubricated forefinger and midfinger of the gloved hand are introduced into the vagina (in many instances only the forefinger can be inserted) (Fig. 18.4). The patient should be told "I am going to place my fingers into your vagina and with my other hand I will be pressing gently on your abdomen." The vaginal walls

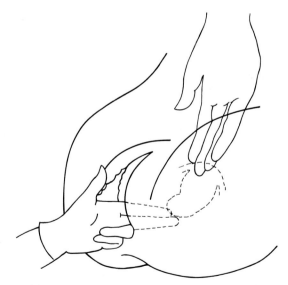

**Figure 18.4.** Bimanual palpation of the uterus.

and cervix are palpated. The position, consistency, mobility, sensitivity, size, contour, and presence or absence of lacerations of the cervix are noted. The normal cervix points toward the posterior vaginal wall making approximately a 45° angle with the vagina.

A genital organs "touch-picture" is gained by palpating the internal genitalia between the hands. The body of the uterus is outlined by pushing the cervix with the corpus uteri upward with the gloved vaginal fingers while the four fingers of the abdominal hands, palpating suprapubically, feel for the fundus of the uterus (Fig. 18.4). The patient should be instructed that "This is your uterus (or womb) and it may feel strange as I move it around." The structures of the anterior abdominal wall are interposed between the examiner's two hands. The size, shape, mobility, consistency, sensitivity, and position of the uterus are noted. The pain elicited by the examination is important. The uterus may be flexed anteriorly or posteriorly and if it is turned back on its horizontal axis, it is said to be in retroversion.

After palpating the uterus, the adnexal regions are palpated. The vaginal fingers are slid into one of the fornices, lateral to the cervix. The abdominal hand is used chiefly to push the adnexa into the pelvis for the vaginal fingers to feel. With experience, one can feel the normal ovary. The ovary is the most sensitive structure in the normal pelvis and the patient should be so advised. It is firm, solid, and moves freely. The normal Fallopian tube is not usually palpable. If a tumor or inflammation is present in these structures, they are more easily palpated. Both sides of the pelvis are examined and compared in this fashion. The perimetrial structures immediately lateral to the cervix are palpated last. They are normally soft, pliable, and insensitive. The chief causes of perimetrial thickening and induration are carcinoma of the cervix and puerperal infection.

Finally, a combined rectovaginal examination should be done. In virgins, a rectal examination may be all that is possible because of the hymen. The patient should be warned "I am going to place one finger in your rectum and leave one finger in your vagina and I will be doing the same motions as before except a little deeper." The middle finger is inserted into the rectum and the index finger into the vagina (Fig. 18.5). Any posterior mass can be felt since only the rectal wall and thin floor of the cul-de-sac separate the palpating fingers. To palpate the perineum, the pelvic peritoneum, or the rectovaginal septum, the index finger is inserted into the rectum and the thumb is placed in the vagina. Using this technique, the patient is asked to strain down while in the standing position to demonstrate a posterior vaginal herniae (enterocele) and differentiate it from a rectocele. Make the patient aware that the exam is nearing the end as these last maneuvers are completed.

Lastly, provide the patient with soft tissues to remove the lubricant from her perineum and genital areas and allow her the privacy for dressing. During this time, write a brief note about your findings and label all specimens that are to be sent for further study. Then review your findings with the patient and allow adequate time for her questions.

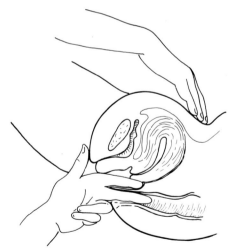

**Figure 18.5.** Bimanual rectovaginal examination.

## Selected References for Further Reading

1. Dumphy, J. E. and Botsford, T. W. *Physical Diagnosis of the Surgical Patient,* 5th Ed. W. B. Saunders, Philadelphia, 1972, pp. 252–269.
2. Fluhmann, C. F. *The Cervix Uteri and its Diseases.* W. B. Saunders, Philadelphia, 1961.
3. Gray, H. *The Anatomy of the Human Body,* 29th Ed., edited by C. M. Goss. Lea & Febiger, Philadelphia, 1973.
4. Huffman, J. W. *The Gynecology of Childhood and Adolescence.* W. B. Saunders, Philadelphia, 1968.
5. Papanicolaou, G. N. The sexual cycle in the human female as revealed by vaginal smears. *Amer. J. Anat. (Supp.). 52:* 519, 1933.
6. Parker, R. T., Parker, C. H., and Wilbanks, G. D. Cancer of the ovary. *Amer. J. Obstet. Gynecol. 108:* 878, 1970.
7. Speert, H. *Obstetric and Gynecologic Milestones.* MacMillan, New York, 1958.

# NINETEEN

# Culture Techniques

Although the laboratory technician usually assumes responsibility for processing material submitted for culture, it is the physician's duty to see that adequate specimens are collected and then delivered promptly to the laboratory. The details of media selection and plating technique are usually determined by the individual hospital laboratory, so this chapter deals exclusively with the methods for obtaining satisfactory clinical specimens.

## GENERAL CONSIDERATIONS

As a general rule, specimens should be collected from a site as close as possible to the suspected source of infection with as little contamination as possible. Equally important is the necessity of withholding antibiotic therapy until the culture specimen is collected. Because the patient plays the essential role of providing the specimen, the physician or nurse must explain how collection is to be done and why the test is needed. A patient who is merely told to "spit in this cup" will never provide suitable sputum for examination.

Swabs should be well saturated or placed within a sterile tube containing culture broth. Swabs that have dried by the time they reach the laboratory are of no clinical benefit. Prompt delivery eliminates the problem of dessication. In order to prevent hazards to laboratory personnel, use sterile containers and try not to spill anything on the external surface.

# BLOOD CULTURE

Blood is perhaps the most important specimen received for bacteriologic examination since any growth reflects a systemic infection which should receive immediate therapy. Great care and judgment must therefore be used when obtaining blood specimens for culture.

Timing is essential because the appearance of bacteria within the bloodstream is characteristically intermittent. There may be as much as a 2-hour interval between the passage of organisms into the blood and the subsequent fever spike (Fig. 19.1). Thus, the folly of the following order, "Call intern to draw blood culture if temperature exceeds 103°." The only way to obtain an ideal culture is to take a specimen in advance of or during the chill, but this is of course not a simple task. If bacteremia is suspected, serial cultures must be drawn. In difficult cases, review the past temperature record for a pattern, and try to anticipate the next fever. Most hospitals maintain

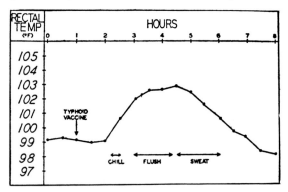

**Figure 19.1.** Typical temperature response of a human being to intravenous injection of a comparatively large dose of typhoid vaccine—100,000,000 organisms. (From *Principles of Internal Medicine*, 5th Ed. edited by T. R. Harrison, R. D. Adams, I. L. Bennett, Jr., W. H. Resnik, G. W. Thorn, and M. M. Wintrobe. The Blakiston Division, McGraw-Hill Book Co., New York, 1966, p. 53.)

a "blood culture tray" which includes syringes, needles, plus the appropriate sterile tubes and broth-filled flasks selected by the bacteriology laboratory. In this way, the blood may be transferred directly to containers at the bedside in order to avoid delay or contamination.

All clinical procedures demand strict aseptic technique but, if there is one that deserves extra care, it is the blood culture. False positive results due to contamination are not only confusing but also prompt inappropriate treatment decisions. A single wipe of the skin with a topical antiseptic is not sufficient. Thorough cleansing with povidone-iodine is to be preferred. Some choose to wear gloves as an added precaution, but many others do not. Allow the prepared skin to dry and draw 10–15 ml of blood. Remove the needle (which may be contaminated from skin contact) before filling the containers. If blood must be injected into a closed container, change needles before doing so. One specimen tube should be provided for detection of anaerobic growth (e.g. thioglycolate broth). Label all tubes with the patient's name, and the time and date of collection. Make certain that specimens are delivered promptly to the lab and placed in an incubator. Blood culture specimens should not sit longer than an hour without incubation.

## URINE CULTURE

The nursing staff is usually responsible for collecting urine culture specimens. One cannot expect to obtain a urine specimen aseptically, except perhaps at the time of laparotomy, because of normal bacteria residing within the urethal meatus. Even when the most cautious technique has been used, bacteria will be found in catheter specimens. Kass has shown that truly infected urine will contain greater than 100,000 organisms/ml. For this reason, hospital laboratories must perform colony counts on urine culture specimens.

Two collection methods may be used: 1) catheterization, a technique which yields the best specimen but which carries the inherent risk of introducing infection, and 2) the clean catch midstream method (the patient is instructed to clean the perineum or penis with soap and then collect only the midportion of the stream). This serves to eliminate resident urethral organisms, which are more likely to appear at the beginning or the end of the stream.

Two final points are worth remembering. The early morning urine specimen is perhaps the best for culture since the urine has had an opportunity to reside in the bladder overnight. Also, the "smegma" beneath the uncircumcised penile foreskin often harbors saphrophytic acid-fast organisms so poor skin preparation may contribute to misleading culture information. Urine cultures must be stored in a refrigerator after collection since urine is an excellent medium for bacterial growth, particularly when left at room temperature before plating.

# NOSE AND THROAT CULTURES

Nasopharyngeal cultures are performed most frequently on infants and children because sputum is so difficult to collect from children. Gently advance a cotton-tipped applicator well into the nostril, twirl the swab 2–3 times, and withdraw. If obstruction is encountered, switch to the opposite side. If there is further difficulty, the nasopharynx can be cultured via the oral route by using a metal cotton-tipped applicator. Bend the tip so that it can be placed above and behind the uvula. Be sure to avoid contact with the tongue upon withdrawal since the oral flora differs significantly from pharyngeal flora.

A throat culture may be performed with a swab and tongue blade. The blade serves two functions; it exposes the posterior pharyngeal wall, and it covers the tongue so the swab will not be contaminated upon withdrawal. If the tonsils are present, run the swab over them and collect any visible exudate. Both nasal and pharyngeal culture swabs should be placed in broth so that they do not dry.

# SPUTUM CULTURE

Satisfactory sputum is perhaps the hardest specimen to obtain for culture. Saliva simply will not suffice. It is the thick mucoid material coughed up from the subglottic respiratory tract which is required for a suitable examination. Patients must be told this for they often equate the words "sputum" and "spit." If they are unable to raise a specimen, then expectorants or saline mist inhalations may be helpful. Satisfactory specimens can often be obtained by inserting a percutaneous transtracheal catheter (Chapter Seven).

Early morning samples are best since bronchial secretions accumulate during the night. The specimen need not be large—2 or 3 ml will do. Examine all specimens before sending them to the laboratory to make sure that sputum is present since it is foolish to waste the lab's time and the patient's money on an inappropriate sample. Remember to ask the lab to perform a smear and gram stain if an immediate choice of therapy must be made.

# CEREBROSPINAL FLUID

At the time of lumbar puncture, 3–5 ml of fluid should be collected aseptically for culture and delivered promptly to the lab. If the fluid is cloudy, ask for a smear and gram stain. Because of the limited volume of spinal fluid, the lab technician should perform the smear so that the culture sample will not be contaminated.

# GENITAL TRACT

When gonococcus is the suspected organism, great care must be taken to obtain a positive smear or culture. Some labs insist that the media be brought to the bedside. A sterile speculum should be used with water as the only lubricant since many of the jellies are antibacterial. Any vaginal exudate is sufficient for the identification of trichomonas but cervical exudate is the best source of gonococci. Immediate smears are most helpful in detecting both trichomonas and gonococci. Urethral discharge can be obtained from the penis for similar cultures.

## WOUND CULTURES

A longstanding tradition calls for habitual use of swab cultures whenever pus is presumed to exist in the confines or vicinity of a wound. Many "uninfected" wounds can produce exudative reactions. Furthermore, swab cultures can never determine the quantitative level of infection present. It can only detect the presence of bacterial contamination.

Many wounds harbor bacterial organisms, particularly open or surface wounds associated with granulating surfaces (i.e. raw surfaces consisting of collagen and proliferating capillaries but without overlying epithelium). Most wounds involve skin which is by definition unsterile. Normal skin flora rarely exceeds $10^3$ organisms per gram. Infection, when applied to wounds, means a quantitative level of infection that becomes a problem (delayed healing) for the surgeon or for the patient, or both.

A significant advance of the past decade is the application of quantitative techniques to wound culture, methods similar to those for urine examination. Quantitative or biopsy wound culture means serial dilution examination of a piece of tissue, about 2 gm (pea sized) taken from a representative wound surface. Don't take fully necrotic tissue. The results may reflect high bacterial counts uncharacteristic of the wound. The actual biopsy should draw blood, proving that the tissue removed lies at an interface with the systemic circulation. Biopsy cultures cause pain, their greatest disadvantage, and their use must be selective and wise.

Specimens are processed by blenderization and then serial dilution. Results are expressed logarithmically as number of organisms per gram of tissue. $10^3$ or less is considered normal.

$10^9$ or greater is considered clinically significant. Wound surfaces with bacterial levels in excess of $10^5/gm$ do not accept skin grafts or endure secondary closure. They may be sources of fever. Patients entering the phase of burn wound sepsis often show bacterial growth at the $10^8$ to $10^9$ level.

Quantitative wound cultures are useful for surveillance of the burn patient whose extent of injury suggests possible development of sepsis. A rise in bacterial count usually precedes systemic signs of infection. Biopsy cultures are also useful as a test preliminary to wound closure, grafting, etc.

Quantitative culture is not useful for identification of organisms present. When this information is needed, a swab culture must also be sent to the microbiology laboratory. A valid qualitative study requires prompt submission of a saturated swab placed temporarily in a tube of broth. Swab cultures can be false negative simply because of dessication or postponed delivery to the laboratory.

Not every wound need be cultured even in the presence of exudate or pus. Remember that incision or drainage of closed infections such as a boil is adequate therapy. Culture sensitivity and antibiotics are needed for diffuse or spreading wound infections.

### Selected References for Further Reading

1. Bailey, R. W. and Scott, E. G. *Diagnostic Microbiology.* C. V. Mosby, St. Louis, 1962.
2. MacDonald, R. A., Levitin, H., Mallory, G. K., and Kass, E. H. Relation between pyelonephritis and bacterial counts in urine. *New Eng. J. Med. 256:* 556–557, 1957.
3. Wood, W. B. The pathogenesis of fever. *Amer. J. Med. 18:* 351–353, 1955.

## TWENTY

# Biopsy

Biopsy, a word coined from "*bios*," meaning life, and "*opsis*," meaning view, literally means a vision of life—an apt definition since the opportunity to view diseased tissue microscopically can provide the physician with a more specific diagnosis. Therefore, opportunities to "view life" ought not to be squandered by careless technique.

During any biopsy, at least two physicians invest their time (the one who takes the tissue sample and the one who examines the tissue microscopically) while the patient invests not only his money but also a certain quantity of physical discomfort. It is, therefore, essential for the operator to obtain the best possible tissue specimen as well as inform the pathologist, either in person or by written word on the request form, exactly what is to be examined and what findings you expect to find. Is there evidence of malignancy in a suspicious and enlarging mole or does this cervical tissue show evidence of estrogen activity? The most capable pathologist works under a tremendous handicap when he is deprived of the clinical information at hand.

## GENERAL PRINCIPLES

Biopsies may be incisional or excisional. The first term implies that the lesion in question is incompletely removed, while the second means that an effort has been made to remove completely the abnormal tissue. It remains for the pathologist to make a judgment regarding the correctness of this assumption.

Incisional biopsies are appropriate when the lesion is large or multiple. For example, a bite biopsy may be taken with an instrument designed for this purpose while performing endoscopic examinations, or a needle biopsy may be obtained from less accessible sites such as the liver. Cell scrapings may be taken for cytologic examinations or a cutaneous lesion may be biopsied with a punch or knife.

The excisional biopsy is commonly performed for individual skin or subcutaneous lesions. These are ordinarily performed as minor surgical procedures in a treatment or operating room, under optimum conditions for cleanliness.

Specimens for permanent section are placed in a fixative (e.g. 10% formalin). Specimens for frozen section should be wrapped in a saline-soaked sponge or towel and delivered promptly to the surgical pathologist. Tissue specimens should not be traumatized since this only produces confusing artifacts. Also remember that the surgeon is responsible for the specimen until it reaches the pathologist. Only responsible messengers should be used, because a lost specimen constitutes negligence in the eyes of the court.

Proper labeling of specimens deserves specific mention. Excisional biopsies, particularly in the presence of malignancy, should be tagged (e.g. with a stitch) and accompanied by a small diagram so that the pathologist may orient the specimen. In this way, the surgeon can be told where positive margins for malignancy lie so that additional tissue may be removed if necessary. If multiple specimens are taken, these must be labeled and *bottled separately*. Multiple rectal polyp biopsies must be identified according to endoscopic level (e.g. 15 cm), so that if one of several is malignant, its site can be known to the surgeon who must plan further resection.

This discussion deals primarily with the various forms of incisional (partial) biopsy, since excisional biopsy truly falls into the category of minor surgery and is discussed extensively in a number of surgical texts.

## SKIN BIOPSY

Adequate specimens of skin may be obtained with a scalpel blade or a 4–6 mm skin punch, designed to cut a cylindrical section (Fig. 20.1). Local anesthesia (1% Lidocaine) is necessary, but care must be taken to inject the drug around and beneath the lesion, *not directly into it.* When cutting an ellipse or cylinder of tissue, try to select a zone at the border of the lesion so that both normal and abnormal tissue will be contained in the specimen. A little bleeding will follow, which usually stops after pressure is applied. Punch biopsies ordinarily leave little or no scar. Elliptical incisions may require a single stitch to bring the skin edges together. This technique is applicable for wound surfaces when quantitative (biopsy) cultures are taken (see Chapter Nineteen).

## ORAL BIOPSY

Areas of either leukoplakia ("white plaque") or frank malig-

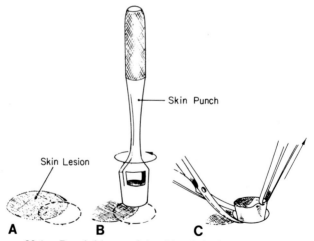

**Figure 20.1.** Punch biopsy of the skin: A, include both normal and abnormal tissue; B, cut cylinder of skin with cutting edge of punch; and C, cut tissue free with forceps and scissors.

nancy within the oral cavity may be biopsied in a manner similar to that described for skin lesions. Patient cooperation and proper illumination are essential. Either a knife or a skin punch may be used. Bleeding can be brisk following oral biopsy so that a catgut stitch might be necessary to achieve hemostasis.

## CERVICAL BIOPSY

Biopsies of the cervix should be preceded by a Schiller test to help to delineate the suspicious areas. Normal cervical epithelium contains glycogen and, therefore, stains dark brown when painted with Lugol's iodine solution. Abnormal cells are devoid of glycogen and, therefore, fail to stain. Poorly stained zones are not diagnostic of cancer, but the test does help to indicate which areas should be examined microscopically. The techniques for cervical biopsies are discussed in more definitive textbooks of gynecology.

## RECTAL BIOPSY

Rectal lesions should be biopsied when found during sigmoidoscopy. Polypectomy, however, should not precede barium enema examination or there is risk of perforation. Anesthesia is unnecessary and bleeding can usually be controlled by applying pressure with a long cotton swab. Rectal biopsy forceps are ordinarily suitable for obtaining a large enough piece of tissue. Removal of the entire polyp requires a snare.

## LIVER BIOPSY

Tissue from less accessible organs, such as the kidney, prostate gland, and liver, may be obtained by percutaneous needle biopsy. A number of needles have been devised for this purpose, but two have achieved popularity and wide use. The Vim-Silverman needle consists of a trocar with two obturators, one solid and the other with two cutting blades designed to cut a core of tissue about 3 cm long and 1 mm in diameter. The Menghini needle is simpler to use and relies on suction force to obtain a specimen.

Liver biopsy remains useful for the diagnosis of a wide variety of hepatic diseases but there are several contraindications. Since hemorrhage is the most frequent and most serious complication, patients with prothrombin times in excess of 18 seconds should *not* be biopsied. A platelet count is also helpful as a screening test. Also, regardless of the laboratory findings, if the skin incision does not stop bleeding within 10 minutes, do not proceed with the needle biopsy. Other contraindications include an uncooperative patient, infection in the right base of the lung, or obstructive jaundice, in which case biopsy may lead to bile peritonitis. Ascites is a relative contraindication, because bleeding seems to be more frequent and severe if the liver is surrounded with fluid.

Liver biopsy should be performed only on hospital in-patients so that they may be observed closely for a 24-hour period following the procedure. Sedate the patient in advance and explain very clearly that he must be prepared to follow directions and hold his breath when asked. Patients with enlarged and easily palpable livers or liver nodules may be biopsied subcostally. Ordinarily, however, the ninth intercostal space in the midaxillary line is the most frequently used site. Following skin prep, anesthetize the skin and interspace with 1% Lidocaine. Then make a small stab wound in the skin with a No. 11 scalpel blade. The technique from this point on varies according to the variety of needle selected.

## Vim-Silverman Needle

Holding the central obturator in place, advance the outer cannula or trocar through the skin and intercostal muscles only. Pause a moment, tell the patient that he won't feel any more pain, and ask him to take a deep breath and hold it until you tell him to breathe. Advance the trocar about three-fourths of its length quickly and remove the solid obturator. Replace it with the forked stylet and advance it completely while the trocar is held stationary, thus placing the blade tips in advance of the trocar tip. Now hold the forked stylet firmly, advance the trocar forward 2 cm over the blades, turn the entire assembly 180°, and withdraw it quickly (Fig. 20.2). If done deftly, the patient should not have to hold his breath more

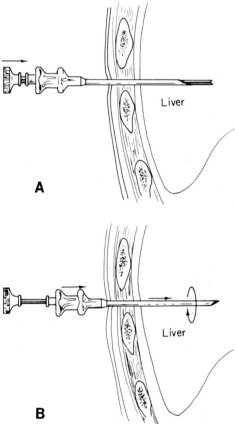

**Figure 20.2.** Liver biopsy with Vim-Silverman needle. A, once the outer cannula is in place, hold it stationary and insert the forked stylet so that the blades advance beyond the needle tip. B, holding the forked stylet stationary, advance the outer cannula over the blade tips, turn both 180°, and remove them quickly.

than 30 seconds. The sequence, however, is very important since it is the advancement of the trocar over the blades which cuts a cylinder of tissue measuring approximately 1 mm × 2–3 cm.

## Menghini Needle

This needle depends on aspiration force and is easier, quicker, and far more dependable. Fix the needle tightly to a Luer-Lok syringe filled with 2–3 cc of saline. Advance it through the skin and intercostal muscles, pause, and inject the saline in order to clear the lumen of the needle. Now pull all the way back on the plunger of the syringe, ask the patient to hold his breath, and advance quickly into and back out of the liver while maintaining constant suction force. After removing the needle, tell the patient that he may breathe. The specimen usually lies within the needle and may be extracted by releasing a little more saline from the syringe.

Both techniques can produce liver lacerations and hemorrhage. The Menghini needle, however, is safer, because it remains within the liver substance for a shorter time interval. If the patient should begin to breathe while a Vim-Silverman needle is in place, release the hub immediately and allow it to move with the diaphragm. Don't grasp it again until the patient is persuaded to hold his breath once more since lacerations are probably the result of diaphragmatic movement while the needle is held rigidly. Patients are asked to remain quiet for several hours after liver biopsy, and periodic vital sign measurement is certainly worthwhile. Routine cross-matching of blood in advance of liver biopsy is not usually necessary since the incidence of intra-abdominal hemorrhage reported by experienced physicians is less than 1%.

# NERVE AND MUSCLE BIOPSY

Numerous systemic neurologic diseases depend on nerve biopsy for their diagnosis, but most physicians are not ordinarily willing to interrupt nerve function for this purpose. One nerve, however, may be removed with little or no sequelae;

namely, the sural in the midposterior calf. It is small and white and readily distinguished.

If necessary, muscle and skin tissue may be obtained at the same time. When excising a wedge of muscle tissue from beneath a layer of well-developed fascia, remember to close the fascia with catgut or else muscle herniation may produce a lump and discomfort afterward. Also coordinate specimen collection with the pathologist who might select special stains requiring no preliminary fixative.

### Selected References for Further Reading

1. Cope, C. and Bernhardt, H. Hook-needle biopsy of pleura, pericardium, peritoneum, and synovium. *Amer. J. Med. 35:* 189–195, 1963.
2. Hardy, J. D., Griffen, J. C., and Rodriquez, J. A. *Biopsy Manual.* W. B. Saunders, Philadelphia, 1959.
3. Menghini, G. One-second needle biopsy of the liver. *Gastroenterology 35:* 190–199, 1958.
4. Moore, G. E. The importance of biopsy procedures. *J.A.M.A. 205:* 917–920, 1968.
5. Vickers, F. N. and Price, D. P. Liver biopsy: a 10-year survey at Louisville General Hospital. *J. Kentucky Med. Assn. 62:* 857, 1964.
6. Wilber, R. D. and Foulk, W. T. Percutaneous liver biopsy. *J.A.M.A. 202:* 53–55, 1967.

# TWENTY-ONE

# Wound Care

During the 16th century, military surgeon Ambroise Pare replied to words of praise with the statement "I dressed him and God healed him." Four centuries later God is still healing wounds, but dressing responsibilities are now discharged by students, and allied health personnel as well as physicians. It seems appropriate, therefore, to devote some attention to the general care of wounds.

## DRESSINGS

Wound dressings were once elaborate affairs because of the prevalent belief that gauze served as an effective barrier to infection. It is now recognized by most authorities that abundant dressings left in place for hours or days are more a source of contamination than a barrier. Since most incisions are sealed by fibrin within a few hours, dressings provide for temporary protection and absorption of secretions. Light dressings are more than adequate for this role and have the added advantage of permitting access to the chest or abdomen for palpitation and auscultation. After the first 24 hours, drainage usually becomes minimal or nonexistent, and initial dressings may even be reduced in size or left off altogether. Some patients will insist on cover since they may be repulsed by the sight of the wound or its stitches.

There are no firm rules about when to change a dressing. Wounds which continue to drain require more frequent attention, perhaps several times each day, whereas incisions which heal primarily may require a change only on alternate days. Dressings which become saturated soon after surgery should *not* be reinforced, but rather changed promptly in order to permit observation of the character of the wound drainage. If dressings have been eliminated altogether, the wound still deserves daily inspection so that complications may be spotted early. There is no rationale for avoiding frequent dressing replacements in order to minimize the risk of cross-contamination between patients. This problem can be minimized only by using appropriate technique, i.e. hand washing, careful disposal of old dressings, etc.

Extremities are best wrapped with an elastic material such as Kling gauze, Kerlix gauze, Ace bandage, etc. Only experience will allow you to know how tight to wrap an extremity, but remember that any patient discomfort calls for prompt revision. Compression dressings should not be limited to the middle of the extremity where they serve as a tourniquet and cause distal edema. Rather, elastic wrapping of any extremity should begin at the toes or fingers regardless of how high the injury is located.

Chronic wounds, i.e. those which because of infection or ischemia heal by granulation rather than by primary intention, deserve special attention. Drainage and bacterial contamination routinely accompany granulation tissue formation. Accumulated pus and necrotic debris must be removed by irrigation with saline until a healthy granulating base develops. Caustic irrigants are not advisable since they do not differentiate between unwanted bacteria and newly formed tissue. Open wounds can be dressed with gauze saturated with a weak sodium hypochlorite (Dakin's) solution. Whenever nurses are involved in wound care they must be given specific instructions and a physician should observe the wound frequently in order to revise the orders when necessary.

Dressings must not only be tailored to the needs of the wound but also serve to protect the surrounding skin. Application of tincture of benzoin around a wound will hold the adhesive tape more firmly as well as guard the skin from abrasive contact with gauze. If dressings are changed several times each day, use Montgomery adhesive straps that may be left on the skin for several days (Fig. 21.1). In the presence of copious drainage, plastic drapes can be used as dressing covers. Retention sutures which are left for 14–21 days often cut into the skin, even though rubber or plastic protectors are used. In order to avoid secondary inflammation from this problem, tuck gauze strips beneath the sutures as they emerge from beneath the skin (Fig. 21.2). Plastic bridges, buttons, and other devices may be used. Finally, remember to obtain periodic cultures during dressing changes on infected wounds.

## SUTURE REMOVAL

The optimum time to remove stitches depends not only on the site of the wound but also on the healing potential of the patient. Wounds about the neck and face heal quickly because of an excellent blood supply, so sutures should be removed early (3–5 days) in order to minimize scars. Trunk wounds usually heal sufficiently to permit skin suture removal in 7–8 days. Abdominal retention sutures ordinarily remain in place 14–21 days. Wounds over moving joints require extra time to heal, and lower extremity wounds need 9–10 days (14 in

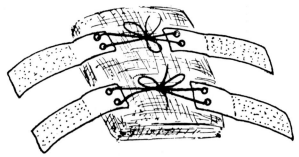

**Figure 21.1.** When dressings must be changed frequently, use Montgomery straps, which may be left in place several days.

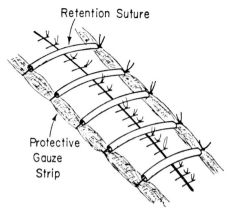

**Figure 21.2.** In order to avoid inflammation when retention sutures cut into the skin, use gauze strips where they emerge from the skin.

patients with occlusive arterial disease) for satisfactory healing. Steroid therapy, uremia, protein starvation, and systemic malignant disease are all indications for leaving sutures in place several extra days.

These are certainly not rigid rules! When in doubt, examine the wound edges before proceeding. If the strength of coaptation appears tenuous, wait 1 or 2 more days. If there is cause for worry after the stitches are already out, then reinforce the incision with adhesive strips or Steri-strips®. However, it is usually a waste of time to remove half of the stitches at a time. Wait until they can all be removed at one time.

When removing sutures, prep the wound with an antiseptic such as Betadine just before starting. Grasp the stitch by its knot, pull slightly, and cut it as close to the skin surface as possible (Fig. 21.3). In this way, suture material which has become contaminated on the skin surface will not be pulled through the sterile tissue beneath. If a wound partially separates after sutures have been prematurely removed, merely approximate the edges with an adhesive bridge. Do not replace the stitches!

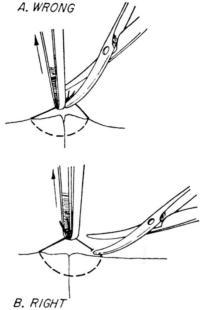

*A. WRONG*

*B. RIGHT*

**Figure 21.3.** When removed, skin sutures should be cut flush with the skin surface.

## DEBRIDEMENT

There are a number of chronic wounds, such as pressure sores, burns, and stasis ulcerations, in which considerable necrotic tissue may accumulate. This tissue not only inhibits healing but also serves as a rich breeding ground for bacterial contaminants. Surgical removal of this necrotic tissue can be carried out at the bedside if the patient is properly sedated and if careful technique is observed. Forceps and dissecting scissors are usually sufficient for the job. A Goulian hand dermatome may be used for tangential excision. Debridement should start in pain-free zones of total necrosis and then progress toward the viable tissue beneath. Excision should stop when either bleeding or pain results. When done properly, bleeding should be minimal, but actively bleeding vessels can be stopped with pressure, by application of thrombogenic material such as Surgicel gauze, or by suture ligature with absorbable material which often must be carried out over a period of several days, rather than in one stage. Always apply gauze moistened with physiologic saline or weak sodium hypochlorite solution after debridement, or dessication will only lead to further necrosis of the newly exposed surface. Topical antimicrobial creams may be used for large open surfaces (e.g. silver sulfadiazine).

# DRAINS

Drains are placed in surgical wounds either to permit the egress of accumulated secretions or to serve as a sentinel for potential complications, e.g. hemorrhage or intestinal perforation. Penrose drains are simple tubes of soft, thin rubber which maintain a drainage route to the skin. Catheters also serve as effective drains since they can be connected to a suction source. Sump drains are special catheters which permit air to be cycled through the lumen in order to provide constant aspiration, and avoid obstruction.

Always remember three important rules about wound drains. 1) Do not remove drains if copious drainage persists. 2) Keep a safety pin fixed to the end of a Penrose drain or suture it to the skin so that it will not recede beneath the wound surface (Fig. 21.4). 3) Do not remove more than 2–3 inches of Penrose drain at one time. If it is removed in one stage, the skin may seal over a functioning tract, perhaps leading to the development of an abscess.

Drains which are left in the gall bladder bed following cholecystectomy course through an 8–9 inch tract. Drainage usually lasts about 2 days, so removal may begin on the second postoperative day and be completed by the fourth. Remove 2–3 inches of drain each day, reattach a new safety pin to the new end, cut off the excess, and reapply a small absorbent dressing. In this way, the drain tract will be encouraged to close from the bottom.

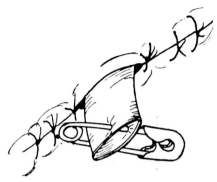

**Figure 21.4.**   A safety pin should be fastened to the end of a Penrose drain at all times so that it will not recede beneath the skin surface. The drain should be sutured to the skin.

Small drains left in breast biopsy or thyroidectomy wounds can usually be removed the morning after surgery. Suction catheters rarely function longer than 48 hours because they become occluded with clot. They should therfore be removed when function ceases, before they become a prime access route for bacterial contaminants. Drains which have been placed as sentinels, on the other hand, must be left in place until after the threat of complication has passed. For example, the Penrose drain left near the duodenal stump during a difficult gastric resection should not be removed until after the risk of perforation has passed (9–10 days).

## STOMAL CARE

Patients with a colostomy, ileostomy, or ileal conduit will eventually learn to care for their own stomas. However, during the early postoperative period, physicians, with the aid of the nursing staff, must provide this service. Most stomal care is directed toward maintaining the integrity of the skin around the stoma. This task is far more difficult for an ileostomy than a colostomy because small intestinal secretions are so much more corrosive. At the completion of surgery, the skin is usually cleansed, dried, and coated with tincture of benzoin. A temporary plastic bag with an adhesive back plate is then applied. The skin should be treated in a similar manner each time that the bag is changed. The hole in the back plate should be no larger than the stoma in order to prevent the bowel contents from coming into direct contact with the skin. In the event of skin inflammation around the stoma, karaya gum, a natural gum resin, is a useful substance available for counteracting the effects of the digestive enzymes contained in bowel contents. Karaya can be placed safely over raw peristomal skin and permits proliferation of healthy skin beneath. It can be mixed as a paste or sprinkled in powder form over raw surfaces. Karaya is not washed away by urine or feces and is rarely allergenic. Ileostomy bag cement even sticks to it! Several types of permanent "ostomy" bags are now available incorporating karaya gum discs which attach to the peristomal skin.

Dilation of stomas is discouraged by most surgeons since more problems than benefits result from this procedure. Also, remember as you provide stomal care to explain to the patient the reasons behind each maneuver. Within a very few days, patients should gradually overcome their fears of the stoma and begin to assume responsibility for its care.

## FISTULAS

A fistula may be defined as any abnormal passage or communication. An unplanned fistula which leads from an internal organ to the skin surface usually produces special wound problems. Most fistulous tracts or sinuses are productive of secretions and require frequent daily dressing changes. Temporary colostomy bags may be useful for any sinus draining large volumes.

Small wound sinuses resulting from a reaction to embedded silk or nylon suture material are perhaps the easiest fistulas to manage. The tract will persist only as long as the irritating stitch remains. A sterile crochet hook is an invaluable aid when extracting sutures from the base of a wound sinus. If this fails, surgical exposure may be required to get all of the iatrogenically placed foreign body out.

Gastrointestinal fistulas, on the other hand, are probably the most difficult of all to manage. Skin problems are far more severe with a high fistula than one located in the lower tract, because of the digestive capacity of the amylase contained in pancreatic secretions. A number of substances have been applied to skin to protect it from pancreatic enzymes, including aluminum oxide paste, peptone beef broth, and even raw meat, which, although impractical, once served as a successful competitive inhibitor of enzyme digestion. Karaya gum, however, takes all the honors for utility and effectiveness and is a sine qua non for the care of any difficult fistula wound. The patient may need to be placed prone on a Stryker frame if the skin becomes too irritated, to permit gravity to drain the noxious fluid away from the skin.

In summary, it is a safe general rule that closely watched and well-cared for wounds do far better than those which are ignored.

### Selected References for Further Reading

1. Connolly, J. E. Prevention of postoperative subcutaneous fluid collection by suction. *J.A.M.A. 157:* 1490, 1955.
2. Dunphy, J. E. On the nature and care of wounds. *Ann. Roy. Coll. Surg. Eng. 26:* 69–87, 1960.
3. Grosjean, W. A. The initial treatment of minor wounds. *Surg. Clin. N. Amer. 36:* 1251–1259, 1956.
4. Harrower, H. W. Management of colostomy, ileostomy, and ileal conduit. *Surg. Clin. N. Amer. 48:* 941–953, 1968.
5. Howe, C. W. Are dressings necessary for abdominal incisions? *Mod. Med. 31:* 280, 1963.
6. Howe, C. W. The bacterial flora of clean wounds and its relation to subsequent sepsis. *Amer. J. Surg. 107:* 696, 1964.
7. Kraissl, C. J. The selection of appropriate lines for elective surgical incision. *Plast. Reconstr. Surg. 8:* 1–28, 1951.
8. Monafo, W. W. Tangential excision. *Clin. Plast. Surg. 1:* 591–601, 1974.
9. Ochsner, A. and DeBakey, M. E. *Christopher's Minor Surgery*, 8th Ed. W. B. Saunders, Philadelphia, 1959.

10. Reid, M. R. Some considerations of problems of wound healing. *New Eng. J. Med. 215:* 753–766, 1936.
11. Rowbotham, J. L. Current concepts: stomal care. *New Eng. J. Med. 279:* 90–92, 1968.
12. Ziperman, H. H. Wound debridement. *Postgrad. Med. 26:* 34–39, 1959.
13. Zovickian, A. Surgery of skin lesions. In *The Craft of Surgery*, edited by P. Cooper. Little, Brown, Boston, 1964, pp. 181–191.

# TWENTY-TWO

# Lumbar Puncture

Lumbar puncture not only serves as an integral part of the complete neurologic evaluation, but also plays an essential role in the induction of spinal anesthesia. This chapter deals primarily with the performance of lumbar puncture for diagnostic purposes, i.e. the collection of cerebrospinal fluid (CSF) and measurement of CSF pressure.

## HISTORY

An American neurologist, Leonard Corning, performed the first spinal tap in 1885, and several reports which followed soon after established the technique as a useful diagnostic aid. During the late 19th century, two Englishmen, Morton and Wynter, described lumbar puncture as a means for relieving increased CSF pressure in cases of severe meningitis. In 1916, Queckenstedt found that he could detect spinal cord tumors by noting an absence of change in lumbar fluid pressure following compression of the jugular vein. This test, which carries his name, is still useful today. During the 20th century, the popularity of lumbar puncture increased following the introduction of regional or spinal anesthesia. The safety of this procedure is now well established and a significant number of children born in the United States are delivered with the aid of spinal anesthesia.

# EQUIPMENT

Spinal trays usually include towels for draping, sponges and prep solution, 10-ml syringe and a 22-gauge (long) needle for local anesthesia, at least three tubes for fluid samples, a three-way valve, a manometer for measuring CSF pressure, and an 18- or 20-gauge by 8.75-cm spinal needle. Anesthesiologists prefer smaller needles (22- or 24-gauge), in order to minimize fluid leakage and decrease the incidence of postspinal headache.

## NEEDED FOR A LUMBAR PUNCTURE:

| | |
|---|---|
| Light | 1% Lidocaine |
| Sponges | Three-way stopcock |
| Prep solution | Manometer |
| Towels | 3 test tubes |
| Sterile gloves | 18-, 20-, 22-, 24-gauge spinal |
| 10-ml syringe | needle |
| 22- and 25-gauge needles | |

# TECHNIQUE

Before starting, it is wise to recall several contraindications to spinal tap. Examine the skin of the back for evidence of infection, in which case the procedure is contraindicated. Septicemia without central nervous system involvement is also sufficient reason to avoid lumbar puncture. Coagulation defects and anticoagulant therapy are relative contraindications; that is, there must be good clinical justification before proceeding in the face of an increased risk of subarachnoid hemorrhage.

The presence of papilledema is also a relative contraindication, since the sudden release of fluid pressure in the lumbar region could result in death following herniation of the brain stem through the foramen magnum. Therefore, lumbar puncture must be preceded by fundoscopic examination. There are situations in which puncture should still be performed in the face of high CSF pressure, e.g. for bacterial identification in the presence of meningitis, but this decision ought to be made by a neurologist or neurosurgeon. Lumbar puncture in the presence of papilledema must be done very carefully with as little fluid removal as possible.

The patient should be positioned correctly or the chance of failure is significant. If he is restless or uncooperative, then assistance will be necessary. Ask the patient to lie on his side, with both knees drawn upward, head flexed, and back arched dorsally. If the physician is right-handed, it is wise to place the patient on his left side and vice versa. The surface of the back must be perfectly perpendicular to the surface upon which the patient rests or the needle might miss its mark (Fig. 22.1). Ask an aide to stand on the opposite side of the patient from you, in order to maintain the patient's position.

Feel for the iliac crest and then palpate the corresponding interspinous space, usually L4–5. (In the adult, the spinal cord extends to the L1 level so any interspace below this is satisfactory.) After locating a satisfactory site, indent the skin with your fingernail so it can be found after preping and draping.

Open the tray, put on sterile rubber gloves, and prep widely, including one interspinous space above and below the preselected site. Apply sterile towels, one on the bed beneath the patient and the other over the iliac crest. If the correct level must be checked again, the crest can then be palpated through the towel without glove contamination.

Warn the patient that he will feel a needle, and then anesthetize the skin with 1% Lidocaine through a small needle (e.g. 25-gauge). It is not necessary to infiltrate the subcutaneous tissue and interspinous ligaments since this will usually inflict greater discomfort than the introduction of the spinal needle will.

Check once more that the patient's back is precisely perpendicular to the bed surface he lies on. Select a spinal needle with

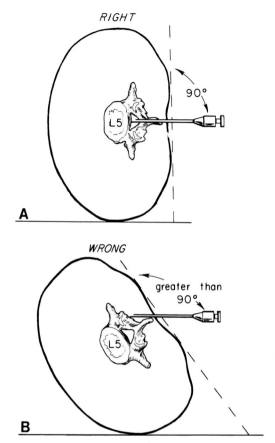

**Figure 22.1.** The needle must be inserted perpendicular to the surface of the back or it will miss its mark. To accomplish this, the patient should be positioned properly.

stylet in place and advance its point into the interspinous space in a slightly cephalic direction. If the needle strikes the spines, withdraw nearly to the skin level and change the direction ever so slightly. Do not intentionally direct the needle away from the midline.

The needle should pass easily through the interspinous ligaments and ligamentum flavum; an experienced hand will feel a small release as the dura is pierced (Fig. 22.2). At this point, remove the stylet and watch for the appearance of spinal fluid. If there is none, turn the needle in case the bevel lies against a nerve root. If success remains elusive, replace the stylet and advance the needle slightly. Firm resistance indicates that the tip has reached the vertebral body. If fluid still fails to appear, then the needle has probably been directed away from midline and shoud be withdrawn almost to skin level and redirected. Persistent difficulty suggests the need to switch to another interspace.

When cerebrospinal fluid appears, attach the three-way valve and manometer and measure the cerebrospinal pressure. Remember that pressure measurements are valid only if the

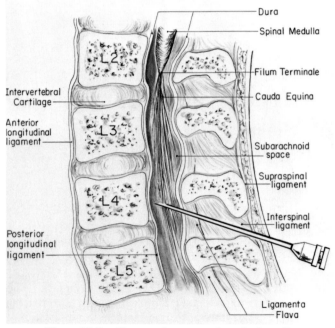

**Figure 22.2.** Correct placement of a spinal needle.

patient is resting quietly. Any unnecessary movement or straining will tend to elevate the pressure. If the pressure is greater than 200 mm of $H_2O$, then collect no more than the fluid within the manometer and send it for routine culture. If the pressure is normal, collect three 2-ml fluid samples in consecutively numbered tubes. Then check the pressure again. The procedure may then be terminated by simply removing the needle.

At the completion of the tap, collected samples should be labeled and sent for culture, cell count, and chemical analysis (e.g. glucose and protein). Remember to write a brief note in the patient's chart recording the character of the fluid, opening and closing pressures, and those laboratory tests which have been requested.

## COMPLICATIONS

Herniation of the brain stem represents the most serious complication of lumbar puncture. Always remember that it is far more easily prevented than treated. In the event of sudden extensor rigidity and respiratory arrest, prompt injection of air may be beneficial, but this complication is ordinarily difficult to reverse. Therefore, in the presence of papilledema, defer action until a neurologist or neurosurgeon can study the risks versus potential gain. Let an expert decide on the need for lumbar puncture.

A less serious but far more frequent complication is the traumatic or bloody tap. This is usually a result of inadvertent puncture of a vein within the paravertebral plexus. Since it is important to differentiate a bloody tap from a recent subarachnoid hemorrhage, observe whether the fluid begins to clear after a few moments. When in doubt, move to another interspace and repeat the tap, or else spin down the fluid in order to determine whether the supernatant is xanthochromic (suggesting subarachnoid hemorrhage) or clear (suggesting recent trauma since there has been no chance for hemolysis).

Headaches may occur following any lumbar puncture, regardless of whether an anesthetic has been administered or not. Their incidence varies from 1–30% and is usually related directly to the volume of fluid lost from the subarachnoid space. Anesthesiologists prefer to use very small needles; e.g. 22- or 24-gauge, in order to minimize fluid leakage and limit the incidence of headache. If a headache does occur, treatment should include supplemental fluid (e.g. 1000–2000 ml either by mouth or by vein).

Other less common complications include meningitis (which almost surely reflects careless technique), inadvertent breakage of a spinal needle at the hub (a result of rough handling), and transitory abducens nerve palsy or hearing loss (which can follow excessive cerebrospinal fluid loss).

### Selected References for Further Reading

1. Cohen, L. A. Lumbar puncture technique in the adult. *GP 29:* 110, 1964.
2. Dripps, R. D. and Vandam, L. D. Hazards of lumbar puncture. *J.A.M.A. 147:* 1118–1121, 1951.
3. Merritt, H. H. and Fremont-Smith, F. *The Cerebrospinal Fluid.* W. B. Saunders, Philadelphia, 1937.
4. Vandam, L. D. and Dripps, R. D. Long-term follow-up of patients who received 10,098 spinal anesthetics. *J.A.M.A. 161:* 586–591, 1956.

# Index

References to figures are in *italics*.

215